Dr Windy Dryden was born in London in 1950. He has worked in psychotherapy and counselling for over 40 years, and is the author or editor of over 200 books, including *Coping with Life's Challenges: Moving on from adversity* (Sheldon Press, 2010), *Coping with Envy* (Sheldon Press, 2010), *How to Develop Inner Strength* (Sheldon Press, 2011), *Coping with Manipulation: When others blame you for their feelings* (Sheldon Press, 2011), *Transforming Eight Deadly Emotions into Healthy Ones* (Sheldon Press, 2012) and *Coping with Guilt* (Sheldon Press, 2013).

Overcoming Common Problems Series

Selected titles

A full list of titles is available from Sheldon Press,
36 Causton Street, London SW1P 4ST and on our website at
www.sheldonpress.co.uk

Overcoming Common Problems Series

Overcoming Common Problems Series

Overcoming Common Problems

Ten Steps to Positive Living

Second edition

DR WINDY DRYDEN

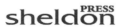
sheldon PRESS

First published in Great Britain in 1994

Sheldon Press
36 Causton Street
London SW1P 4ST
www.sheldonpress.co.uk

Reprinted seven times
Second edition published 2014

British Library Cataloguing-in-Publication Data
A catalogue record for this book is available from the British Library

ISBN 978–1–84709–270–0
eBook ISBN 978–1–84709–271–7

Typeset by Caroline Waldron, Wirral, Cheshire
First printed in Great Britain by Ashford Colour Press
Subsequently digitally reprinted in Great Britain

eBook by Fakenham Photosetting Ltd, Fakenham, Norfolk

Produced on paper from sustainable forests

I dedicate this book to the memory and legacy
of Dr Albert Ellis and Dr Arnold Lazarus.
Their ideas have had a powerful influence
on the development of my own thoughts about positive living
and have helped shape this book

Contents

Preface

Of all the books that I have written for Sheldon Press, this is perhaps the one of which I am most fond. This is not because it is the best selling of all my Sheldon books, although it is; nor is it because it is the book that many therapists recommend to their clients as an introduction to the theory and practice of Rational Emotive Behaviour Therapy (REBT), the therapy upon which the book is based. I am most fond of this book because it expresses in succinct and accessible form the ideas that underpin psychological health and because of the way that it was put together.

The first edition of this book was written in 1993 and published in 1994. Actually, strictly speaking, I did not write the book in 1993, I dictated it in 1993. For I spoke the book into a mini-cassette recorder every day during a two-week period while walking down Madison Avenue in Manhattan from my friends' house – where I was staying on East 93rd St – to the Albert Ellis Institute on East 65th St. My then assistant, Caroline Dearden, transcribed these recordings and I worked on the transcript and put it into publishable book form.

As I made clear in the first edition, the ten steps presented in this book are not perfectly sequential. I suggest that you take Steps 1–6 before Steps 7–10. However, feel free to use this book in whatever way makes sense to you.

While the first edition of the book has stood the test of time and I am still basically happy with it, like any sturdy structure it required a makeover, some internal reorganization and some modernizing. I have performed these activities and I hope that the second edition is as well received as the first. As ever, I would be grateful to receive any feedback that you care to give. Your comments should be addressed to me c/o Sheldon Press.

Windy Dryden, London and Eastbourne

Step 1

Assume personal responsibility

I begin this book with a discussion of personal responsibilty and urge you to assume responsibility only for what you are, in fact, responsible for.

What are you personally responsible for?

The concept of personal responsibility is a major feature of mental health. The former Chief Rabbi, Dr Jonathan Sacks, once said that you are responsible for matters which are within your sphere of influence, and I very much agree with him. Just what, then, are you able to influence in your life? The prime areas that you are able to influence are those that belong to you as an individual. By this I mean your thoughts, your feelings, the decisions that you make and the way you act. You also have *some* influence over the likely consequences of your actions.

Not that you are in perfect control of any of these. For example, if you desperately try to control your thoughts you will soon learn that you are unable to do so. Try this experiment. Close your eyes for a moment and think of a pink elephant. Now instruct yourself that you must not think of a pink elephant. You will find, much to your surprise, that the one thing you cannot dispel from your mind is a pink elephant. However, if you allow yourself to think of a pink elephant, you will soon become bored with this thought and your mind will wander on to other things. This experiment shows that you have some control, but not perfect control, over your thoughts. Your thoughts fall, broadly speaking, within your sphere of influence and therefore you are responsible for them. Nobody else is responsible for them. For example, I am not responsible for you thinking of a pink elephant, even though I am responsible for inviting you to think of it. My invitation is within my own sphere of influence and therefore I am responsible for it.

In other books I have written for Sheldon Press (e.g. *How to Accept Yourself*, 1999; *Coping with Envy*, 2010; and *How to Develop Inner Strength*, 2011), I have shown that your feelings largely depend on your beliefs about yourself, other people and the events that you experience in your life. This means that you are responsible for the feelings that you experience. Since you are largely responsible for the beliefs that you hold about yourself, other people and the world, you can be said to assume the major responsibility for the feelings that stem from these beliefs. You do not have total control over your beliefs or your feelings because you will encounter adversities that will influence the beliefs that you hold and the feelings you experience. However, despite this influence, you still have a fair measure of control over what you believe and what you feel in the face of these adversities.

For example, let's suppose that you enjoy the company of close friends, but your job has taken you away to another country where you do not know anybody. You are experiencing an adversity, which is a negative activating event. Being in this situation, therefore, has some bearing on the way you are going to think, given your desire to be with people that you know and love. Since you are facing an adversity, it is unlikely that you will think, 'Good. I'm pleased that I am away from my close friends', or 'It doesn't matter to me one way or the other that I am cut off from the people I care about.' Indeed, it would be unhealthy for you to think in such ways. However, facing this adversity does not absolve you of your responsibility altogether for the way you think about your plight. You will have a choice between holding a rational belief, e.g. 'I don't like being in this situation but I can stand it', and holding an irrational belief, e.g. 'I can't stand being in this situation, I'll go crazy if I have to put up with it for another moment.'

The events that you experience in your life, particularly negative events (what I call adversities in this book), do restrict your choices of how you are going to think, but they rarely *cause* the way you think and feel. You almost always have a choice of thinking rationally or irrationally.

You are also largely responsible for the decisions you make in life, even though you may not have all the information you need when you make a decision. Imagine, for example, that you have been offered two jobs. You are unemployed and you are faced with making three choices. First, you could take job A. Second, you could take job B. Or, third, you could choose to remain unemployed and wait for a better job to come along. (Here, of course, you are taking the risk that you will not find a better job.) It is your responsibility to find out as much as you can about the two jobs that have been offered to you and also about the chances of finding a better job if you decide not to take either of them. Let's suppose that you decide to take job A. It quickly transpires, however, that important information was withheld from you which, had you known about it, would have meant that you would have made a different decision. You are still responsible for making the decision that you took, but you are not responsible for the fact that important information was withheld from you. It would be counter-productive for you to demand that you should have known this information when the reality was that you didn't know it. This is an important point: you are not responsible for knowing what you did not know. While you cannot be held responsible for something that you didn't know at a given moment, you are responsible for learning from this experience. Thus, next time you could ask certain questions about a job that you didn't ask about job A.

You also have some responsibility for the likely consequences of your actions. Imagine that you have made a promise to do something for a friend. However, when the time comes for the favour, something more interesting crops up and you decide not to keep your promise. It is very likely that your friend is going to be displeased that you did not help him in the way you agreed. Here, it can be said that you are responsible not only for your failure to keep your promise (i.e. your action) but also for the disappointment of your friend. However, you cannot be held responsible for your friend's feelings of severe depression, since his depressed feelings stem largely from the disturbed way that he was thinking about your failure to keep your promise. So, if your friend accuses you of making him depressed, he is wrong: while you are responsible for breaking your promise to him, he is largely responsible for his feelings of depression.

What all this means is that it is very important for you to take responsibility for your thoughts, feelings, decisions and actions, and for the likely consequences of these actions. Unless you assume personal responsibility, you will not strive to change what you can change; rather, you will tend to blame other people or life events for the way you think, feel and act and for the decisions that you make. Blaming other people and external events for what you are really responsible for is a hallmark of poor mental health. When you do this, you tend to see yourself as a victim and take an 'I am helpless', self-pitying view towards life. Refusing to accept personal responsibility means that you also refuse to take control of your life. As such, you look towards others to rescue you and become overly dependent on them. Being a victim you will tend to complain bitterly about your lot and how unfairly you have been treated by others and by the world.

If you do this you will tend to blame your past and your parents for the way you think, feel and act today. Unfortunately, some schools of psychology tend to reinforce this by not distinguishing between past events *contributing* to the way you think, feel and act today, and those same events *causing* your thoughts, feelings and behaviour. My view is that your past certainly has an influence, but it can rarely be said to cause the way you respond to life events now. The way you respond now depends largely upon the beliefs you hold about current and future events. You may have learned from your parents, for example, that if you fail to do well in life this means that you are a failure. However, don't forget that in all probability you have spent many years keeping this philosophy alive in your own head. Thus, my view is that you are responsible for choosing – yes, choosing – to keep alive these philosophies and that you can learn to change them.

Responsibility is different from blame

It is very important to distinguish between responsibility and blame. While I am arguing that people are responsible largely for the way they think, feel and act, it does not therefore follow that they need to be blamed for their thoughts, feelings and actions and the consequences of their decisions and actions. For blame involves the beliefs that others must not behave badly, that they are bad people if they do bad things and that they need to be punished for so doing. What I argue in this book is that people are fallible human beings, neither good nor bad: when they do something bad they need to take responsibility for it, but they do not have to blame themselves for their wrongdoings. As I have shown in my book *Transforming Eight Deadly Emotions into Healthy Ones* (Sheldon Press, 2012), blame stops you learning from your errors. If you are to be blamed, this means you are a bad person, and if you are a bad person you will continue to do bad things.

To summarize, take responsibility for what is within your sphere of influence, but do not take responsibility for what is not within your sphere of influence, particularly for what is within the sphere of influence of others. When you take responsibility for your thoughts, feelings and actions, doing so will encourage you to change your unhealthy thinking patterns which are linked to your self-defeating emotions and self-defeating behaviours. If you assume the responsibility that you undoubtedly have, you will be able to benefit from the rest of the book. If you continue to deny this responsibility, then it is unlikely that you will benefit from this or any other self-help material that you may purchase.

Step 2

Adopt flexible beliefs about your desires

As I have shown in Step 1, your feelings and behaviour are largely dependent upon the way you think about the events in your life. Thus, if you are to be mentally healthy, it is important that you develop a set of beliefs and attitudes which enable you to do so. I call this set of beliefs and attitudes a philosophy. In my view, a mentally healthy philosophy is essentially flexible.

A model of human emotions

What constitutes a mentally healthy, flexible set of beliefs, and how does this differ from a set of beliefs that is rigid and will lead to poor mental health? I can best answer this question by teaching you a model of human emotions which I regularly teach my clients in the course of counselling them. This model has three parts.

Part 1

I want you to imagine that you believe it is desirable or preferable for you to have a minimum of £11 with you at all times. You do not believe that it is essential to have this sum with you at all times, just that it is preferable. Imagine, then, that you are holding this flexible belief as you check how much money you have in your pocket or purse. You discover that you only have a £10 note. How do you think you would feel about having £10 when you desire, but do not insist on, having a minimum of £11 with you at all times? I think you will see that you would feel concerned or disappointed. These negative emotions are, I argue, healthy because they enable you to adjust to this negative situation and motivate you to take constructive steps to correct the situation, if it is possible for you to do so.

Part 2

Now I want you to imagine that you are holding a different belief. This time you believe strongly that you absolutely *must* have a minimum of £11 with you at all times. This is essential and it would be the end of the world if you didn't have this sum. With this belief clearly in mind, how would you feel about only having £10? I think you will see that you would have an entirely different set of negative emotions: those which are unhealthy. For wouldn't you feel anxious or even depressed? These emotions are hardly likely to encourage you to adjust to the situation, nor would they help you to take constructive action to try to remedy it.

Now, please note that in Parts 1 and 2 of the model you are facing the same situation, i.e. you have £10 in your pocket. Note also that your very different negative emotional reactions – in the first part a healthy set and in the second part an unhealthy set – stem from different philosophies. In the first part, you were holding a flexible, non-demanding philosophy, while in the second part I asked you to hold a rigid, demanding philosophy.

Part 3

In this final part of the model, I want you to imagine that you are still holding the same rigid, demanding belief that I invited you to hold in the second part, namely that it is absolutely essential that you have a minimum of £11 with you at all times and it would be terrible if you didn't. Now imagine that while desperately searching in your pocket or purse, you find two £1 coins that you didn't realize you had. How would you feel about having £1 more than you believe you need? Most people say that they would feel relieved, and for a while you probably would too, because you have discovered that you have more than your absolute minimum. However, while you were still holding the rigid belief: 'I absolutely must have a minimum of £11 with me at all times and it would be terrible if I didn't', one thought would occur to you which would lead you to feel anxious again. You may begin to think along the lines, 'What if I lose £2, what if I have to spend £2, or what if I get robbed?' Once again you will be in a state of anxiety, even though you now have more than your absolute minimum.

The point of this model – and this is a very important point and one that I really want you to think about – is that human beings, whether they be rich or poor, male or female, black or white, young or old, make themselves emotionally disturbed when they don't get what they believe they must have and are vulnerable to emotional disturbance when they do have what they believe they must have because they could always lose it. However, if human beings stick rigorously (not rigidly!) to their non-dogmatic, flexible beliefs, then they will experience negative emotions if they don't get what they want, but these negative emotions will be healthy and help them to adjust to the situation and encourage them to take constructive actions to try to change the situation.

The importance of keeping your desires flexible

As a human being, you live your life according to a complex set of desires. You want certain things to happen and prefer other things not to happen. You have preferences for yourself: you want certain things from other people and you have a healthy set of wants and wishes in relation to the world in which you live. As the above model shows, as long as you keep your preferences flexible and non-demanding, then you will be emotionally healthy even if you do not get what you want. As I will show you later in the book, certain negative emotions are healthy responses to situations when your desires are not met. This non-demanding, flexible set of preferences, wishes and wants helps you to change what you can change and adjust constructively to what you cannot change about your life, without making yourself emotionally disturbed in the process. These desires also encourage you to take constructive action which is directed towards fulfilling your desires. Thus, these non-demanding, flexible beliefs related to your desires and preferences encourage you to strive towards personal happiness and positive living.

However, when you take your desires and make them rigid by saying that they are absolute necessities, musts and 'have tos', then two things happen. First, you increase the likelihood that you will experience emotional disturbance when you don't get what you demand that you must get, and you increase your vulnerability to emotional disturbance even though you may have what you demand you must have. Second, when you hold rigid beliefs, you act in ways that decrease your chances of getting what you want in life. As the model shows, anxiety largely stems from rigid beliefs about threat, and you are unlikely to act constructively when you are anxious. When you are anxious, it is as if you are running around like a headless chicken, trying unthinkingly and desperately to find its head. Is the headless chicken a good model to encourage you to take constructive action? Of course not! However, if you hold a set of flexible rather than rigid beliefs, you will experience healthy negative emotions like concern and sadness – as opposed to anxiety and depression – which are designed to help you not only acknowledge the reality of the situation you are in, but also stand back and think constructively about how you can change the situation, if in fact it can be changed.

Different human beings have different desires, and it is not my job to tell you what your desires should be. For example, you may have a desire for love and approval, or to make your mark in life and achieve high status. You may have a desire to be in control, or for fairness to exist in the world. All of these desires are healthy as long as you put the word *but* after them. Thus, if you want to be loved, it is healthy for you to say, 'I want to be loved by a significant other, *but* I do not have to have this love.' If you desire fairness, it is healthy to believe, 'I want to see fair treatment in the world and I will strive to help to bring this about, *but* there's no absolute law that the world must act according to the principle of fairness.' It is when you take the *but* out of your desires that you transform your flexible desires into rigid and demanding musts. This inflexible, rigid philosophy is at the core of emotional disturbance and leads you to be vulnerable to that disturbance even if you have what you believe you must have in any given situation.

So, if you want to be mentally healthy, it is important for you to recognize what your desires are, to strive to achieve them and to problem-solve your way out of situations which frustrate you in your pursuit of these desires. Moreover, if you refrain from transforming these desires into rigid, inflexible demands and musts, you will remain mentally healthy. However, if you insist on escalating your desires into absolute, rigid musts, then you will always be at the mercy of poor mental health.

There are three main reasons why your rigid and demanding philosophies are irrational. First, as long as you demand that you must get what you desire, then, as the model shows, you will get poor emotional and behavioural results in life. Second, rigid musts are inconsistent with reality. If, in fact, there was a law of the universe that stated that you must get what you want, then the world would have to operate according to that law and give you what you want, no matter what. Since it is obvious that no such law exists, then rigid, demanding musts are irrational in that they do not accord with the way the world is. Third, your demands and musts do not logically follow from your healthy preferences. Ask yourself this question: would you like, right now, £1,000 to drop into your lap? You would probably answer 'Yes' to that question. However, does it logically follow that because you want £1,000 to fall into your lap, therefore it absolutely has to? Obviously not! Therefore, musts are irrational because they do not logically follow on from your preferences.

Teach your children well

In this step, I have made the point that a flexible belief is a belief where, when you hold it, you assert what you truly want, but you do not demand that you have to have it, whereas when you hold a rigid belief you believe that you have to have what you want. I have found that my clients really understand this distinction once they have imagined teaching it to a group of children. Let me start by outlining how you might teach children about flexible beliefs (sometimes called non-dogmatic preferences).

Children, as you live your life you will have many desires. You will want certain things to happen and you will want other things not to happen. Don't be ashamed of what you want or wish for. Being aware of your desires is a very important part of being human. However, as important is learning the following lesson:

Just because you want something to happen does not mean that it has to happen. And just because you want something not to happen doesn't mean that it mustn't happen.

Sometimes you get your desires met and sometimes you don't. And because you don't always get what you want and sometimes get what you don't want, it is important that you develop an attitude that reflects this fact of life. The best way of doing this is for you to keep in mind two important points that you need to combine into one belief: acknowledge that you want something, but also accept that there is no law that dictates that you have to get what you want.

Let me show you how to do this with respect to one of your desires for something to happen. Let's suppose that you want to go to university when you grow up. There is, of course, nothing wrong with this desire, assuming it is something that you truly want for yourself and not something that you don't want but are doing for other people. This desire will motivate you to work hard for something that is important to you. However, just because you want to go to university, it doesn't follow that it is essential for you to get this desire met. You don't have to go to university, even though it is important for you to do so. While at first glance it might seem that this component will stop you from trying to get into university, this isn't the case. It will, in all probability, stop you from being anxious and won't interfere with your striving to get what you want. Thus, your desire will motivate you, and your realization that it isn't essential to get what you want will help prevent you from being anxious as you work to achieve your goal.

So, children, to sum up: acknowledge what you want, strive for it if it is in your best interests to do so and accept that, just because you want something, it doesn't mean that it is essential for you to get it.

Now, let me outline how you might teach children about demands.

Children, as you live your life you will have many desires. You will want certain things to happen and you will want other things not to happen. When your desires are strong, you will be tempted to believe that it is absolutely necessary to have these desires met. Give in to this temptation. Convert your desires into absolute necessities. Tell yourself that because you want something to happen, it has to happen. And tell yourself that because you want something not to happen, it must not happen.

Let me show you how to do this with respect to one of your desires for something to happen. Let's suppose that you want to go to university when you grow up. If this is important to you, tell yourself not only that you want to go to university, but that you have to go to university, it is absolutely essential for you to do so. Now there is a downside to converting your desires into absolute necessities and you should be aware of this downside before deciding whether or not to convert your desires into demands. Your desire to go to university will motivate you to work hard for something that is important to you. If you convert this desire into a demand and believe that you must go to university no matter what, you may work even harder and do so to the exclusion of everything else. You may even get obsessed about going to university. On the other hand, when you convert your desire into a demand, you may get anxious and this may stop you from working productively on your studies. This is the price that you pay for converting your desires into demands.

So, children, to sum up: acknowledge what you want and convert your strong desires into demands. You run the risk of becoming emotionally disturbed if you do so, but this can't be helped.

You now know the difference between a flexible belief (or non-dogmatic preference) and a rigid belief (or demand). Which of these two principles would you choose to teach to your group of children?

Hopefully, the answer is obvious.

Step 3

Accept reality and keep the horror out of badness

In striving to become mentally healthy, it is very important for you to develop an accepting attitude towards reality and to keep horror out when that reality is bad. Let me first discuss what I mean by accepting reality.

Accepting reality

Whenever I talk about accepting reality, people mistakenly think I am encouraging them to resign themselves to reality. However, this is far from what I mean. 'Resignation' implies that there is little or nothing that you can do to change what exists. Therefore, if you are feeling resigned to a situation, you do not make the effort to change it, with the result that the situation does not change. So let me make it crystal clear that I am not encouraging you to resign yourself to life's adversities and I do not wish to discourage you from taking constructive action – far from it. By accepting reality, I mean that you acknowledge that a situation exists, because all the conditions are in place for it to exist, and that you also make constructive attempts to change these conditions and thereby to change the situation.

When I encourage people to accept reality, some think that I am encouraging them to like reality or to become indifferent to it. This is, again, far from what I mean. Let's suppose that you have applied for a job that you would really like to get. However, your application is rejected. If I were to encourage you to accept the reality of your rejection, I would not be suggesting that you should like being turned down for the job. This is unrealistic, because for you to like the rejection you would have to hold the rather strange belief, 'I am pleased that I have been turned down for a job that I really want to get.' Nor am I encouraging you to be indifferent towards the job rejection. This would be stoicism taken to the extreme. In order for you to be indifferent towards your job application rejection, you would have to believe something like, 'It doesn't matter to me one way or the other that my job application has been rejected.' This would clearly be a lie!

Accepting reality in this example means that:

- you acknowledge the fact that your job application has been turned down, for reasons as yet unknown;
- you actively dislike this situation since it is against your desires;
- you consider whether or not to challenge the decision of the appointments panel.

On this latter point, you may decide to contact a member of the panel to discover the reasons for your rejection. If you are given a reason which you consider to be unfair, you might decide to invite the panel to reconsider its decision. Here you are trying to do something to modify the conditions that were in place and that led to your job rejection. However, just because you are attempting to change those conditions does not mean that you will be successful. The likelihood is that even if you are told the reasons for the appointment panel's decision, you may not be successful in getting them to reconsider their decision.

So, accepting reality, in general, involves three major steps:

- You acknowledge that the situation does exist and that all the conditions are in place for it to exist.
- You acknowledge that the existing situation is against your desires and that you actively dislike it.
- You decide whether or not to take constructive action to try and change the situation.

Incidentally, if your attempts to change the situation fail, accepting this reality would mean acknowledging that your attempts to modify the situation were unsuccessful and that this too is unfortunate.

Awfulizing and the importance of taking and keeping horror out of badness

Being human means that you will have a large number of desires. Some of your desires are going to be mild, some moderate and some strong. As a rule of thumb, the greater your desire, the more negative you will feel if your desire is thwarted. It is usually when your strong desires are not realized that you may find it difficult to follow the above three steps and may hold instead an awfulizing belief.

Awfulizing beliefs

When you hold an awfulizing belief, you do the following. First, you acknowledge that it is bad that you have not fulfilled your desire. Second, you irrationally believe that this situation absolutely should not exist. Third, you conclude that because what absolutely should not have happened has in fact happened, it is not only bad, it is more than 100 per cent bad. It is literally horrible, terrible and the end of the world.

This awfulizing belief is virtually always a grossly exaggerated negative evaluation. Here, you begin by rating negative events on a 0–99.99 per cent scale of badness. Then you invent a totally new scale of horror which goes from 101 per cent badness to infinity. When you hold an awfulizing belief, you believe, at that moment, that nothing could be worse. If you stand back and reflect on this idea for a moment, you will quickly see how ludicrous it is. You are literally, in common parlance, getting things way out of proportion.

How to take and keep the horror out of badness

In order to change your awfulizing belief you need to take and keep the horror out of badness. You can do this by taking the following steps.

First of all, you need to ask yourself for evidence in favour of your rigid belief that this negative event absolutely should not exist. I hope you can see that if something exists, unfortunately all the conditions are in place for it to exist. If you demand that it absolutely shouldn't exist, you are failing to accept reality. You are, at bottom, demanding that reality absolutely should not be reality, that what exists absolutely must not exist. This is as sensible as demanding that when two parts of hydrogen are mixed with one part of oxygen, they absolutely should not make water. I hope you can see that when H_2 is added to O, what exists is water because all the conditions are in place for water to be produced. Demanding that adding H_2 to O should not make water has no effect whatsoever on the production of water under these conditions. In the same way, when something has happened to you, like a job rejection, demanding that this should not have occurred isn't, in itself, going to change your job rejection into a job offer. Indeed, the more you demand that this situation absolutely should not exist, the more disturbed you will be, and if you decide to try and change the situation when you are emotionally disturbed it is likely that you will make things worse by antagonizing the appointment panel, which won't encourage them to give you a fair hearing.

Second, you need to challenge your idea that the situation you do not like is more than 100 per cent bad. Many years ago, Dr Albert Ellis, the founder of a therapeutic approach called Rational Emotive Behaviour Therapy, was talking about awfulizing beliefs to an audience and claimed that being run over by a steamroller is 100 per cent bad in that nothing could be worse. A member of his audience quickly corrected him, saying, 'Dr Ellis, even being run over by a steamroller is not 100 per cent bad because you could be run over by that steamroller more slowly!'

My erstwhile American colleague Dr Tom Miller had a novel way of helping people to rethink their awfulizing beliefs. Let's suppose that you consider being rejected from your desired job to be awful, meaning more than 100 per cent bad. Dr Miller would encourage you to develop a different scale against which you can compare the badness of your job rejection. Let's suppose, he would argue, that having all four of your limbs cut off is, for the sake of argument, 100 per cent bad. He would then ask you to rate lesser situations: having three of your limbs cut off might be 90 per cent, two limbs cut off 80 per cent, one limb 70 per cent and so on, right the way down to a situation where you might rate a permanent scar on your face as being 5 per cent bad by comparison, and a scar which heals to be 1 per cent bad. Dr Miller would then ask you whether your job rejection was as bad as having four limbs cut off. Would it be equal to having three limbs cut off? Two limbs? One limb? And so on. I have used his technique with many people and very few of them opt for a job offer in exchange for a permanent scar on their face. Although this technique may seem bizarre at first sight, it does help you to get things in proportion in a way which is quite vivid and dramatic.

I hope that I have conveyed the message to you that when you hold an awfulizing belief, you are making a grossly exaggerated negative evaluation of something which is certainly bad, but is not nearly as bad as you think it is when you are in the grip of your awfulizing belief. As the mother of Smokey Robinson (the Motown singer and songwriter) told her son: 'From the day you are born till you ride in the hearse, there's nothing so bad that it couldn't get worse.'

Teach your children well

I have made the point that in order to be mentally healthy it is important that you take the horror out of badness, and contrasted this belief with an awfulizing belief where you transform badness into horror. I have found that my clients really understand this distinction once they have imagined teaching it to a group of children. Let me start by outlining how you might teach children about non-awfulizing beliefs.

> Children, as I have told you, in life you will have many desires. I have explained to you that it is important that you do not transform these desires into necessities and that you do not demand that you must get what you want. This will help you to respond constructively when you don't get what you want. When this happens, it is important that you learn this second lesson:
>
> *When you don't get what you want and you don't demand that you have to get it, consider this situation to be bad, unfortunate, but not the end of the world, terrible or awful.*
>
> When you hold a non-awfulizing belief you acknowledge that something can always be worse and that good can come from not getting what you want. Thus, when you want to go

to university but do not demand that you must do so, you acknowledge that it would be bad if you did not get into university, but you recognize that far worse could happen to you and you also realize that if you failed to get into university, it would be possible for you to turn this to your advantage.

So children, to sum up: when you want something, but do not demand that you have to get it, remind yourself that it is bad when you don't get what you want. However, keep in mind that it isn't awful not to get what you want and that worse could happen to you. Also, remember that good can come from not getting what you want.

Now, let me outline how you might teach children about awfulizing beliefs.

Children, I have already said that when your desires are strong, you will be tempted to believe that it is absolutely necessary to have these desires met. I urged you to give in to this temptation and convert your desires into absolute necessities. When you do so and you don't get what you believe you must get, tell yourself that it is the end of the world, terrible or awful.

When you hold an awfulizing belief you acknowledge that nothing can be worse and that no good could possibly come from this situation. Thus, when you believe that you must get into university, you will tend to think that it would be awful if you don't and that you could not possibly turn this to your advantage since nothing good could possibly come from this state of affairs.

So children, to sum up: when you demand that you have to get what you want, remind yourself that it is the end of the world when your demand is not met, that nothing could be worse and no good could possibly come from your unmet demand.

You now know the difference between a non-awfulizing belief and an awfulizing belief. Again, which of these two principles would you choose to teach to your group of children? Again, hopefully the answer is obvious.

Are tragedies and unfairness awful?

There are, of course, adversities which would score very highly on any scale of badness that we could construct. Personal tragedies do happen: you may, in fact, lose a limb; you may tragically lose a loved one through death or even violence; you may lose all of your possessions and your house in a fire. I certainly do not wish to encourage you to minimize the tragic nature of these events. However much we may wish for a world where such tragedies do not happen, such a world is, in all probability, not going to exist. Accepting reality under these conditions means that you acknowlege that (a) tragedies can and do happen to you; (b) you are not immune from such tragedies and neither do you have to have such immunity; and (c) tragedies are very bad and may have a lasting impact on you. By contrast, when you hold an awfulizing belief about your tragedy, you are, in fact, demanding that such a tragedy *must* not happen to you. Is there any law of the universe that provides you with immunity from such tragedies? I hope you can see that you do not have any personal immunity from the tragic events that I have outlined and, in addition, there is no law of nature that decrees that you must have such immunity. If there were, tragedies could not possibly happen to you. Thus, even when tragedies happen, it is very important that you do not add emotional disturbance to the strong negative emotion of sadness, which is a healthy response to these tragedies. I am not minimizing the badness of any tragedy, I just wish to encourage you to accept the tragic nature of reality and to refrain from holding an awfulizing belief about tragic events.

We live in a world where tragedies happen and where unfairnesses exist, and no matter how undeserving you are of unfair treatment, this does not mean you are immune from it and neither does it mean you have to have such immunity. Accepting the reality of life's unfairness involves you taking the following steps.

First, it involves you giving up the demand that because you do not deserve to be treated unfairly, such an unfairness must not exist. Second, it involves you acknowledging that, unfortunately, the conditions that led to the unfairness did in fact exist at the time and, in an empirical sense, should have existed, in the same way that adding H_2 to O should make water. Third, it involves you rating the unfairness on a realistic scale of badness, being mindful that when you reach 95 per cent or above this is equivalent to the tragedies that I have already outlined or having three or four limbs amputated. Fourth, it involves you trying to change the unfair situation if you can, or to gracefully accept (but not like) it if you cannot change it.

Accepting the realities of change, uncertainty and complexity

Whatever attitude we take, there are three facts of life that we would be wise to accept. First, change happens whether we like it or not. Second, we often face uncertainty in life, partly because we cannot predict the changes that will inevitably happen in life. Third, the world we live in is complex, and as changes continue to occur it is becoming more complex.

Accepting change

It is a truism that we live in a world where change constantly occurs. Even as you read these words you are in a process of change and flux. Also, other people constantly change and so do your relationships. When you make demands that you, other people and the world you live in must remain the same and that change must not occur, you are failing to accept reality. Holding such a non-accepting belief will not alter one iota the fact that change will occur. Change occurs whether or not you demand that things must stay the same. Isn't it more mentally healthy to accept this without disturbing yourself about it? Do you remember the story of King Canute? He thought that he was all-powerful and thus he stood in front of the advancing tide and commanded it to go back. What happened to King Canute? He got his feet wet. Why? Because the tide came in whether or not King Canute made demands on it to go back!

Accepting uncertainty

You may refuse to accept reality and thereby make yourself mentally unhealthy when you demand that you must have certainty in your life and conclude that it would be awful if such certainty failed to exist. However, if there is any certainty in this world, it is that there is no certainty. Why? Because things change, often in ways that you cannot predict. Thus, to demand that you must have certainty in your life does not in any way bring about such certainty. Indeed, when you demand certainty and add horror to the mix, you still face uncertainty, but you do so with emotional disturbance. Isn't it more mentally healthy to accept that uncertainty is the human condition and not to disturb yourself about it, even though you might healthily prefer certainty to exist? Of course it is. So give up your demand that certainty must exist, accept (but do not like) uncertainty and keep horror out of this unfortunate state of affairs.

Accepting complexity

You may have a preference for life events being clear-cut, which is fine as long as you do not transform your preference into a demand. For, if you do make such a transformation, you will put events into two categories, either black or white. Unfortunately, the world and life conditions are far less clear-cut than this. You just cannot fit the complex nature of life experiences into two discrete categories. If you try to do this you may end up like the guests of Procrustes.

Procrustes owned the equivalent of a modern-day hotel and insisted that his guests had a comfortable night's sleep. He believed that they had to fit his bed exactly, otherwise he was sure they would not be comfortable. So what did Procrustes do? He cut off the legs of those who were too tall for his bed and stretched the bodies of those who were too short. When you demand that things must be unambiguous and clear-cut, you think and act as Procrustes did. Unfortunately, the one who suffers is you. The world does not become clear-cut just because you demand it be so. In what was perhaps a fitting end to his nefarious activities, Procrustes fell victim to his own black-and-white way of viewing the world. Hearing of Procrustes' 'hospitality', Theseus (later famous for killing the Minotaur) anticipated his host's move and made Procrustes lie in one of his own beds, first decapitating him so that he would fit perfectly! While you will not come to such a gruesome end if you demand that life be clear-cut, you will, in all probability, lose your head emotionally!

Another non-accepting attitude you may hold that leads to emotional disturbance and that relates to your failure to accept the complexity of life is the demand to be right. If you hold such a belief, you may think that there is a right way of doing something, a correct attitude to hold or a proper way of looking at things, and that other people have to share your view. This attitude will frequently get you into enormous difficulty with other people, as Edward de Bono showed in his accurately titled book *I am Right, You are Wrong* (Viking, 1990). This is because you find it intolerable when other people disagree with you and you cannot accept that there may be different and equally valid opinions about an issue. This dogmatic attitude is at the root of fanaticism and terrorism.

In reality, life cannot be divided up into such clear-cut, right–wrong categories. There are different ways of looking at the same issue. There are different and equally legitimate views that people take towards the same event. In short, pluralism exists in the universe and it is clear that in the vast majority of the fields of human endeavour universally accepted views do not exist. To accept the reality of pluralism you need to acknowledge that you have a particular view which you consider to be right, but that there are different views which other people are entitled to hold. If only fanatics and terrorists could accept this reality, think how much safer the world would be.

Adopt a non-Utopian outlook

Finally, to accept reality you need to adopt a non-Utopian outlook. Here, you acknowledge that negative and positive events exist in the world. You avoid adopting a naive Pollyanna-ish optimism where you assume that the future is bound to be bright and there will be no clouds on the horizon. You also avoid taking an over-pessimistic view about the future where you assume that things are bound to be negative and that there will be no positive events on the horizon. If you adopt a non-Utopian philosophy, you will focus on and try to maximize the positive aspects of reality and also recognize and try to minimize the negative aspects of reality. In short, a non-Utopian outlook recognizes that the world is a mixture of good and bad rather than all good or all bad.

Step 4

Develop a greater tolerance for discomfort

Introduction

As a human being, you are constantly faced with making decisions which have implications for your short-term and long-term interests. When you make a decision which helps you to meet both your short- and long-term goals, then you normally have no difficulty at all in making this decision. It is when your short-term interests conflict with your long-term interests that problems start. I believe that mental health involves striving to achieve a constructive balance between your short-term and long-term goals. If you constantly put off trying to meet your short-term goals in pursuit of your long-term goals, you may well experience very little pleasure in life. However, if you constantly strive to meet your short-term goals and neglect your long-term goals, you may feel comfortable in the moment, but you will frequently conclude that your life is rather shallow and uninteresting. Striving to achieve a healthy balance between your short-term and long-term goals gives you a sense that you are pursuing personally meaningful goals and provides you with a reasonable level of immediate comfort.

From my long experience as a counsellor, I believe that one of the hardest things for people to do is to work towards their long-term goals while putting up with short-term discomfort. Why is it that we find it so difficult to forgo immediate pleasure or comfort when doing so would help to enrich and enhance our lives? The main reason is that we frequently act according to discomfort intolerance beliefs. If this applies to you, you may:

- frequently procrastinate;
- lead an undisciplined lifestyle;

- frequently fail to persevere at tasks that it would be in your best interests to stick with;
- go out of your way to avoid the hassles of life, despite the fact that dealing with these adversities would increase your chances of living more resourcefully.

You may find that your unpaid bills mount up as you push them aside, believing that out of sight is out of mind. In addition, if you hold discomfort intolerance beliefs, you may find that you seek out quick fixes for your problems. Thus, you may overeat, over-smoke, drink too much, gamble too much and try to shop away your blues.

If you recognize yourself in the above description, it is very likely that you go to your preferred comfort zone whenever you experience discomfort. I have written a book for Sheldon Press on this very subject (*How to Come Out of Your Comfort Zone*, 2012).

Major discomfort intolerance beliefs

So, what are some of the major discomfort intolerance beliefs that you are likely to hold?

'I must be comfortable now'

A major discomfort intolerance belief is the idea that you must be comfortable in the moment and that it would be unbearable if you were to be uncomfortable. Having achieved a state of comfort, if you believe this idea you will fight tooth and nail to cling to it and will certainly not be prepared to make yourself temporarily uncomfortable, even if doing so is in your best interests.

Imagine that you are sitting in a very comfortable chair and you know that you have washing-up to do in the next room. If you believe that you must be comfortable now, it may take heaven and earth to move you out of your comfortable armchair. You will move when it becomes more uncomfortable for you not to do the washing-up. You still believe that you must be comfortable, it is just that doing the washing-up suddenly becomes more comfort-able for you than leaving it. If you have such a need for comfort, you will constantly be motivated to seek the most comfortable option available to you, even though doing so will lead you into greater trouble in the longer term.

'I must not be frustrated'

A second major self-defeating discomfort intolerance belief is the idea that you absolutely must not be frustrated, and if you do experience frustration in your life then you cannot tolerate it. With this belief, when you are faced with frustration, your first and often only thought is to try desperately to get rid of it by whatever is the quickest means at your disposal, even though this may increase your frustration in the future. However, since your only concern is ridding yourself of frustration *now* you really do not care that you are setting yourself up for more trouble in the future.

'I must not experience negative feelings'

If you believe that you must not experience negative feelings and that doing so would be unbearable, two things are likely to happen. First, you will go out of your way to avoid situations in which you are likely to have negative feelings, even though these negative feelings may well be healthy, and even though allowing yourself to experience them may lead to greater satisfaction later. If you do this, your life is dominated by the principle of avoidance and you will sense that you are leading a very restricted life. If only, you exclaim to yourself, the world was a nicer place and if only people could be nicer to me, then I might venture out. Because you believe that you cannot stand negative feelings, you will not only refuse to take healthy risks, you will also overestimate the amount of negativity that there is in the world. Also, it never occurs to you that it is possible to confront negative events and live through them. Your only thought is not to experience negativity.

Second, your intolerance of negative feelings may well increase the pain of these negative feelings when these are unavoidable. This commonly occurs when you bring this idea to your experience of anxiety. You then believe that you must not be anxious and that you literally couldn't stand it if you became anxious. This 'anxiety about anxiety' will literally lead you to escalate your anxiety into blind panic.

These two manifestations of the idea that you cannot stand feeling negative often go together. Thus, you live your life according to the principle of avoidance whenever possible, but you may also escalate your anxiety into panic because you can never completely eradicate negativity from your life and certainly not from your own imagination!

'I must experience good feelings'

The fourth major discomfort intolerance belief can be phrased thus: 'I must experience good feelings and life would be unbearable if I wasn't constantly happy, joyous and having pleasure.' If you believe this idea, your life will be characterized by one of a number of self-defeating patterns. First, you may become addicted to one of the many substances or activities that characterize those with an addictive personality. You may try to get a good feeling by drinking alcohol, eating chocolate or taking marijuana, heroin or cocaine. You may become addicted to gambling or you may get your kicks from constantly shopping. The problem with all these activities, of course, is that the effects only last for a short period; you will then need another dose of the 'pleasurable' substance or activity fairly soon after the effects of the previous dose have worn off. If you do not identify and work hard to give up the idea that you must always experience pleasure, it could literally kill you.

You may develop a less dangerous style of life as a consequence of believing that you must experience good feelings, i.e. you may be constantly and easily bored. If you demand that you must only experience good feelings you will focus on the negative aspects of even pleasurable activities. For example, Simon, who likes to play tennis, believes that he must only experience enjoyment in life. Before going on to the tennis court he is enthusiastic because he has a false image in his mind. He assumes that the entire experience will be pleasurable. However, his enthusiasm soon wanes because, even though he enjoys tennis, there are certain frustrations involved with the game. If he is not playing against somebody who is just above his level, he quickly becomes bored, particularly if his opponent is less talented than himself. He also quickly becomes discouraged if he plays somebody who is more talented than him since he is easily beaten. Furthermore, Simon becomes disenchanted with the fact that he has to collect the tennis balls from the net and he also gets easily frustrated when his opponent throws the ball inaccurately to him when it is his turn to serve. People like Simon can literally never be satisfied since even the most pleasurable of activities have some frustrating aspects. The Simons of this world, because of their attitude, focus on these negative aspects, demand that they shouldn't be there, exaggerate them in their own mind and rob themselves of satisfaction.

Procrastination: a major consequence of discomfort intolerance

I hope you can see now that if you hold one of the four beliefs mentioned above – 'I must be comfortable', 'I must not be frustrated', 'I must not experience negative feelings' and 'I must only experience good feelings' – you will easily tend to procrastinate. Procrastination, literally translated, means putting off until tomorrow what it would be wise for you to do today. If you procrastinate, you will easily invent what you consider to be good reasons for not starting the work that you need to do today. However, if you are honest with yourself, you will see that these 'good reasons' are really excuses or rationalizations. Some of these rationalizations include the following:

- 'I need to be in the mood in order to start the work.' This is blatantly untrue because frequently you can start the work when you are not in the mood and get into the mood as a result of doing the work!
- 'I need to be under pressure or I need to be keyed up in order to do the work.' This again is not true. If you procrastinate you may indeed only work when you are under pressure because at some point it is more uncomfortable to procrastinate than to do the work. However, it does not follow that you need to be anxious or under pressure in order to start the work. If you started the work earlier when you were not under pressure, you could give yourself much more time for creative thought and do a better job as a result.

If you procrastinate, you may do so because procrastination has a built-in excuse. If you don't give yourself enough time to complete a task and you don't do it well, you can always attribute your poor performance to the fact that you didn't have enough time to do it. This spares you from recognizing that you may have gaps in your knowledge or skills that you need to improve. Since you defend yourself against such threatening information with the excuses that you make, you rarely learn from your experiences.

Improve your level of discomfort tolerance

What does it take for you to raise your level of discomfort tolerance and live a more mentally healthy existence? The first and most important aspect of developing discomfort tolerance beliefs is for you to challenge the rigid beliefs that underpin discomfort intolerance.

Challenging your demands about discomfort

In order to do this you need to become aware of when you are seeking comfort, when you are avoiding frustration, when you are avoiding situations in which you might feel negative or when you are engaging in self-defeating activities in order to feel good in the moment. The next step is to look for the following types of attitudes:

- 'I must be comfortable.'
- 'I must not be frustrated.'
- 'I must not experience negative feelings.'
- 'I must feel good in the moment.'

Then you need to challenge such attitudes again and again by asking yourself three questions. First, and most importantly, ask yourself: 'Does this belief lead me to live a more effective, mentally healthy existence or will it get me into significant trouble with myself and other people with whom I come into contact, and will it sabotage my long-range goals?' I hope I have shown you that discomfort intolerance beliefs will almost inevitably lead to poor results in the longer term.

Second, you need to ask yourself, 'Is there a law of the universe that exists which proves that I must be spared discomfort, frustration or negative feelings, or proves that life conditions must be arranged to make me feel good?' Such laws only exist in your head; the universe does not follow along these lines. If the universe really did operate according to your demands, then you would constantly be spared frustration, you would constantly be comfortable, you would constantly not feel negative, you would constantly feel good, and you would be spared any negative consequences as a result of achieving these states. Unfortunately, the world does not operate according to your desires, and as long as you believe that you must be spared frustrations, etc., you will continue to defeat yourself. By all means stick with your healthy preferences about gaining comfort, avoiding frustration and so on, but don't transform these into rigid demands. Your healthy preferences will help you to achieve such states in constructive ways, but will also help you to bear in mind that it is important for you to come to a healthy compromise between achieving your short-term goals and achieving your longer-term goals.

Finally, you need to ask yourself, 'Does it logically follow that because I prefer not to be uncomfortable, therefore I absolutely must not be uncomfortable?' Again, a moment's consideration will help you to see that this is a poor logical conclusion: musts do not logically stem from preferences.

You need to challenge these ideas again and again and, most importantly, you need to act on your new healthy, flexible beliefs. Thus, while challenging the idea that you must not be uncomfortable, you need to act according to the idea that discomfort is undesirable but that it is necessary to put up with it if you are to achieve more meaningful goals. There is no law which states that you must not be uncomfortable. Such discomfort is, unfortunately, a fact of life. Believing this will help you to problem-solve your way out of the frustration situation, if this is possible.

Raising your level of frustration tolerance involves a paradox. Changing your philosophy of low frustration tolerance and acquiring a philosophy of high frustration tolerance is a frustrating and uncomfortable venture. But if you show yourself that it is worth tolerating, then you can do it.

Challenging your discomfort intolerance beliefs

The second major belief that you need to focus on and change is the belief that discomfort, frustration, negative feelings or the absence of positive feelings is unbearable and you literally cannot stand it. This means two things. First, it means that you will literally drop dead if you do experience frustration, for example. Second, it means that you can never experience any happiness again for the rest of your life if the frustration is allowed to exist and cannot be eradicated immediately. I hope you can see that such situations rarely, if ever, exist and that you can stand what you think you cannot stand.

You need to ask yourself the same three questions about the 'I can't stand it' philosophy as you did about your rigid beliefs. First, is believing that you cannot stand discomfort going to help you to live more effectively or is it going to sabotage you? The latter is almost always true. Second, is there a law of the universe that states that you cannot stand discomfort, etc.? If there is, you won't be able to stand it under any circumstances even if it means saving the life of a loved one. Putting it into that context, I hope you can see that the idea that you cannot bear discomfort, for example, is literally nonsense. Finally, you can ask yourself: does it logically follow that because discomfort is difficult to tolerate, it is therefore impossible to tolerate? Again, this is an arrant overgeneralization.

In order to change your 'I can't stand it' belief to one which states 'I don't like it, but I can stand it', you need to challenge your discomfort intolerance beliefs again and again and act according to your alternative discomfort tolerance beliefs until these become more habitual for you.

Teach your children well

Again, you may find it easier to grasp the important differences between discomfort intolerance beliefs and discomfort tolerance beliefs by imagining yourself teaching the differences to a group of children. Let me start by outlining how you might teach children about discomfort tolerance beliefs.

Children, I have explained to you about the importance of keeping your desires flexible and not transforming them into rigid demands. If you do this, you will learn a third lesson:

When you don't get what you want and you don't demand that you have to get it, you will find this bearable although it may well be a struggle for you to bear it, especially when your strong desires have not been met. However, it will frequently be in your interests to bear this state of affairs.

When you hold a discomfort tolerance belief you acknowledge that you will neither die nor disintegrate if your desires aren't met, nor will you lose the capacity for future happiness. Thus, if you want to go to university, but do not demand that you must do so, you acknowledge that not going would be difficult for you to bear, but that you could bear it and it would be in your interests to tolerate it. You can thus experience happiness in the future if you don't go to university.

So, children, to sum up: when you want something but do not demand that you have to get it, remind yourself that not getting what you want is bearable and worth bearing even if it is a struggle for you to put up with the deprivation.

Now, let me outline how you might teach children about discomfort intolerance beliefs.

Children, I have already told you about converting your strong desires into demands. When you do so and you don't get what you believe you must get, you will probably tell yourself this state of affairs is intolerable.

When you hold a discomfort intolerance belief you believe that if your demand such as going to university is not met then this is unbearable and you will never be happy again, or you will disintegrate or even die.

So, children, to sum up: when you demand that you have to get what you want, you will also tend to believe that you can't bear it if your demand is not met.

You now know the difference between a discomfort tolerance belief and a discomfort intolerance belief. Once again, which of these two principles would you choose to teach to your group of children? I hope the answer to this question is self-evident.

Developing a greater tolerance of discomfort is one of the most important – and sadly one of the most neglected – topics in the psychology of mental health, and I have therefore discussed it at length. For further information and details of techniques on developing a greater tolerance for discomfort, see my book *How to Come Out of Your Comfort Zone* (Sheldon Press, 2012).

Step 5

Develop a healthy attitude towards yourself

There are many popular psychology books that help you to develop more successful and caring relationships with others. There are far fewer texts designed to help you to have a better and more caring relationship with yourself. Yet the relationship you have with yourself frequently affects the relationships you have with others and with the world in general. As Albert Ellis, the famous American psychologist, has put it: if you cannot be helped to live comfortably and at peace with yourself, how can you hope to live in harmony and effectively with others? So, in this section of the book, I will cover the important ingredients that go to make up a mentally healthy attitude towards yourself.

Unconditional self-acceptance

The first important ingredient involves you developing an unconditional self-accepting attitude. It will undoubtedly surprise many of you to learn that I am against the concept of self-esteem. Why? If you define self-esteem carefully, you will see what I mean. First of all, what is the self? I agree with my friend and colleague Dr Paul Hauck, who says, in his book *Hold Your Head Up High* (Sheldon Press, 1992), that the self is made up of our characteristics, thoughts, feelings, behaviours, interests and other features. In order, therefore, to esteem yourself, which really means giving your 'self' a global rating, you need to know everything about yourself from the moment you are born to the moment you die. How can you gain an accurate record of all the above aspects, since there will be billions and billions of them? Also, what is the purpose of giving yourself such a global rating? Is it so that you can get into heaven or make the downward journey into hell? It certainly cannot be to improve your mental health, since for you to be a worthwhile person, everything about you would need to be worthwhile. I hope that you can see that this is impossible to achieve: human beings are, by essence, fallible, which means that we can and do make mistakes and that we are a complex mixture of the good, the bad and the neutral.

Another reason I am against the concept of self-esteem is that it is normally conditional. By this I mean that you consider yourself to be a worthwhile (or a more deserving person) as long as certain conditions exist. These conditions may include acting competently, winning the love of significant individuals, acting morally and so on. When you consider yourself to be a worthwhile (or more deserving) individual for as long as these conditions exist, you are vulnerable to making yourself miserable if the conditions change. Therefore, if you are a more worthwhile person because you have acted morally, it follows that you are a less worthwhile person for acting less morally. In this, you are also making an overgeneralization. You begin with the healthy and useful evaluation of one of your acts (i.e. 'It is bad that I acted immorally') and then you overgeneralize by making a global rating of your total 'self' (e.g. 'I am bad for acting immorally'). Here, you are also giving yourself a label which is not warranted by a specific act or even a series of acts.

If you hold a belief based on conditional self-esteem, even when you consider yourself to be a worthwhile person – for acting competently, for example – you are still anxious underneath, because in order for you to maintain your worth, you need to continue to act competently. Being a fallible human being, you will always make mistakes and act less competently, and thus as long as you make your self-esteem conditional upon competent actions, you are always vulnerable to underlying anxiety and other emotional disturbances.

There are two major alternatives to conditional self-esteem which will give you much better emotional results and help you to lead a more mentally healthy life. The first is what is called unconditional self-esteem. Here, you still insist on giving yourself a total rating (which has its problems, as discussed above) but your self-esteem is based on conditions which are not going to change.

Thus, you may consider yourself to be a worthwhile person simply because you are alive. If you develop this belief, you will live a mentally healthy life, and if you believe in an afterlife then all you need to do is to renew your decision to consider yourself to be worthwhile as long as you are alive in your next life! Alternatively, you can consider yourself to be worthwhile as long as you are human. Since it is very unlikely that you will ever perfect yourself or become inhuman or a robot in your lifetime, this position will also work.

Both of these positions, however, are philosophically problematic. Somebody may come along and say, 'Well, I consider you to be worthless because you are alive', or 'worthless because you are human'. Your decision to consider yourself worthwhile because you are alive or because you are human is therefore based on an act of faith. If you are prepared to make such an act of faith, fine. You will be able to live a mentally healthy existence for as long as you are able to sustain this belief.

The second, more challenging but I believe more realistic and rewarding position is for you to refrain from giving your 'self' a global rating at all. Here, you recognize that you are far too complex as a human to be given a single rating, and that if you were to so rate yourself you would be making an arrant overgeneralization and giving yourself an unwarranted label. Instead, you accept yourself as a fallible human being who is complex and has good, bad and neutral qualities. Doing this will help you to maximize your good qualities and strive to minimize, although never eradicate, your negative qualities. Please realize, though, that you will never be able to master this self-accepting philosophy fully. Why? Because you are human and as such you have an in-built predisposition to make unwarranted generalizations and, under certain conditions, to jump very easily from rating an aspect of yourself to rating your total self. Realistically you can strive to minimize (rather than eliminate) your self-rating tendencies and to maximize (rather than perfect) your self-accepting tendencies.

I mentioned in Step 1 of this book that acceptance does not mean resignation and I wish to reiterate this point here. When I encourage you to accept yourself as a fallible human being, I am not – repeat *not* – encouraging you to resign yourself to who you are in the sense of not working to change aspects of yourself which are self-defeating and to maximize those aspects of yourself which are self-enhancing. I believe that adopting a self-accepting philosophy encourages you to work towards changing yourself. It does not lead to a discouraged, resigned state.

Teach your children well

Again, you may find it easier to grasp the important differences between depreciation beliefs and unconditional acceptance beliefs by imagining yourself teaching the differences to a group of children. Let me start by outlining how you might teach children about acceptance beliefs.

Children, here is the fourth and final lesson that I want you to learn:

When you don't get what you want and you don't demand that you have to get it, if your thwarted desire is down to your own behaviour you can rate your behaviour negatively without rating yourself negatively. Rather, you can accept yourself as a complex, unrateable fallible human being whose behaviour is negative. If your thwarted desire is down to someone else's behaviour, you can accept him, for example, as a fallible human being who has acted badly. And if your thwarted desire is down to life conditions you can rate these conditions negatively without depreciating the whole of life.

So, if you really want to go to university, but do not demand that you have to go, you will:

1 accept yourself, but dislike your behaviour if you were primarily responsible for your failure to get to university;
2 accept others, but dislike their behaviour if they were primarily responsible for your failure to get to university; and
3 accept life, but dislike the specific set of life circumstances that were primarily responsible for your failure to get to university.

So, children, to sum up: when you want something but do not demand that you have to get it, you will accept yourself, others or life for whoever or whatever is responsible for you not getting your desire met.

Now, let me outline how you might teach children about depreciation beliefs.

Children, I have already told you about converting your strong desires into demands. When you do so and you don't get what you believe you must get, you will tend to depreciate yourself if you were responsible for not getting your demands met, depreciate others if they were responsible for you not getting what you believed you must get, or depreciate life if life conditions were responsible for not gratifying your demands.

So, if you demand that you have to go to university, you will:

1 depreciate yourself if you were primarily responsible for your failure to get to university;
2 depreciate others if they were primarily responsible for your failure to get to university; and
3 depreciate life if a specific set of life circumstances were primarily responsible for your failure to get to university.

So, children, to sum up: when you make demands, you will depreciate yourself, others or life for whoever or whatever is responsible for you not getting your demands met.

You now know the difference between an acceptance belief and a depreciation belief. Finally, which of these two principles would you choose to teach to your group of children? For the last time, your answer should be self-evident.

Celebrate your individuality

Part of being human involves acknowledging that you are a *unique* individual. Never again will there exist a person with your constellation of traits, abilities, strengths and weaknesses. When I lecture on how to develop a healthy attitude towards oneself, I tell my audience that in all probability there will never again exist an individual who has my mixture of interests. For example, I am keenly interested in soul music, particularly in the records of Junior Walker and The All Stars. I also love the songs and recordings of Al Jolson and I am a keen Marx Brothers fan. I support Arsenal Football Club, delight in reading Billy Bunter books and am an avid writer on psychotherapy and emotional self-help. I doubt very much that you will ever meet another individual with this combination of interests. Given this fact, I can choose either to celebrate my individuality or to consider myself a freak and an odd-bod. I prefer the former because it is healthier, it is more consistent with reality and it represents a more logical and realistic approach to life. I thus invite you to consider the myriad ways in which you are a unique individual and to celebrate your own individuality.

When I was much younger I believed that there were certain interests that I absolutely should have and certain interests that I absolutely shouldn't have. Thus I believed, in an absolute sense, that I *should* enjoy the works of William Shakespeare and classical music, and that I *shouldn't* enjoy watching soap operas and professional boxing on the television. In doing so, I learned to deny my own individuality and became ashamed of having certain interests. Now I do neither. I firmly believe that as long as an interest is absorbing for you and doesn't cause harm to other people, animals or the environment, then there is nothing wrong with having that interest even though other people may frown on you for having it. Thus, if you enjoy train spotting, do not let the sneering attitudes of others deter you from pursuing that hobby. If you get a kick out of playing tiddlywinks, fine: go and pursue it. Discover, if you can, like-minded individuals who share your idiosyncratic preferences and enjoy them with such people. Do not fall prey to the idea that you absolutely *shouldn't* have certain preferences because such a view is inconsistent with reality, illogical and ultimately self-defeating. Allow yourself to have the interests and the preferences that are truly yours and pursue them energetically.

Also, celebrate your unique constellation of traits. Know and understand what your personality characteristics are and seek out environments in which you can express these characteristics and avoid, as long as it is not self-defeating to do so, environments which constrain the expression of your characteristics. This is especially important when choosing a career, vocation or occupation. If you are an extrovert, for example, it may be preferable for you to avoid jobs which are not going to allow you to express that trait (e.g. an accountant, civil servant or museum curator). Likewise, if you are basically introverted, you will probably not be happy in vocations that demand a high level of extroversion such as acting, selling and other vocations which involve you making an immediate personal impact. While there are, of course, exceptions to these rules, I believe it is important for you to know your personality traits and characteristics and make a reasoned decision about those environments which will allow you best to express them.

If you are in doubt on this point, you may find it useful to consult one of the reputable career counselling agencies to help you discover the vocations which will enable you to express your unique constellation of personality traits (and, of course, interests).

Develop an attitude of self-care

Unless you can find somebody who will put your interests above his or her own, it is important, and a sign of mental health, that you do this for yourself. Indeed, if you do find somebody who is willing consistently to put your interests above her own, you may be in for trouble. Such a person is likely to have a very poor opinion of herself, may tend to be exceptionally needy and will do anything to please you. Ultimately you will find having a relationship with such an individual over-restricting and claustrophobic.

I am not suggesting that you be selfish – far from it, for selfishness means cynically putting yourself first all the time, while disregarding the interests and desires of others with whom you are involved and expecting them to fit in with your narcissistic and selfish way of life. What I mean by an attitude of self-care (also known as enlightened self-interest) is that you basically look after your own interests while realizing that, as you are involved in relationships with others, it is important that you also strive to ensure that you honour your commitments to them and have their interests in mind. By self-care, I do not mean that you will always put yourself first and others a close second. Indeed, you may at times choose to put other people's interests above yours, particularly those of your children, who did not ask to be brought into the world by you. Even here, expert opinion has it that children flourish when they perceive that their parents healthily look after their own interests and do not subordinate their interests to those of their children. So the essence of self-care is flexibility. You are basically caring for yourself and looking after your own interests: not in a selfish way, so that you ignore the interests of others, but in a way that is flexible and is responsible to the demands of different situations.

A large part of self-care is the development and maintenance of healthy boundaries. As a human being, you need to look after yourself physically (I will discuss this point later in this step). You also need to care for yourself emotionally and to set aside time for healthy and solitary reflection. As you are involved with a number of significant others, it is healthy to take this fact of life into consideration. Furthermore, you will, in all probability, have to work for your living and therefore you need to discharge your responsibilities to your employers. Additionally, you may have hobbies and interests and undertake voluntary work. If you do not set healthy boundaries and limits between all these activities, you may very easily find yourself overwhelmed and may end up in a situation where your physical and emotional well-being is at the bottom of the pile, together with your desire for solitary reflection.

What I am advocating, then, is that you consider, in the service of your mental health, all your responsibilities and activities and plan to spend time in each of these areas. This, of course, means that you need to think carefully about your priorities and allocate sufficient quality time and quantity time to those responsibilities. To do this, you will need to use time effectively, which is another hallmark of being an emotionally healthy individual.

Consider one of my clients, Alex. He stated that in his life his wife and children have the highest priority, but when I investigated how much time he spends with them as compared to the time he spends with his friends, on his leisure activities and on his work, he was shocked to learn that his family only justify a small fragment of his time. He believed, as unfortunately a lot of people do, that because he has a caring attitude towards his family, this attitude is enough and he doesn't have to spend time with them. What I helped Alex do was to reorganize his life so that he spent time in a way which reflected his priorities and his values. This meant that he chose to forgo certain activities which he found pleasurable and to limit the time he spent on others. In the long run, Alex considers himself to be a happier, healthier individual, yet it was only when he learned to allocate his time according to his values and to draw healthy boundaries around all of his activities that he had a chance to experience the happiness which actualizing one's values brings.

It is a truism to say that we only have one life, yet many people conduct themselves as if they expect to live several times over. 'I'll make time for this later,' they say. If you are such a person you will often be confronted with the discrepancy between your stated priorities and the way you actually live your life, notably at those times when you come face to face with your own mortality (e.g. when you discover that you are overly stressed or experiencing a life-threatening illness). How many times have you read about people who have said that having an illness has helped them to step back and rethink the direction of their lives? You don't need to experience such a potentially life-threatening situation in order to consider what your priorities are, to draw healthy boundaries around all your responsibilities and activities, and to choose to live life according to your stated values and preferences. Think about it.

Honour your commitments to yourself

Numerous people are at risk of putting other people and activities before themselves. They may have certain plans – for example, to write a novel or to go travelling. They may even commit themselves to these plans, but how often do they honour their promises to themselves in the sense of taking action in line with their commitments? Again, how many times have you heard people say, 'If only I had an opportunity to live my life over again, I would have done such and such differently'? I don't wish to sound morbid, but it may be useful to imagine that you are lying on your deathbed.

What 'if onlys' are you saying as you lie there? Make a note of them and plan to honour your commitments to yourself while you are able to do so. Avoid the 'if only' trap and accept the grim reality, which is that you may not be able to do everything you want to do in this one life that you have. Prioritize your activities. Accept the fact that the items that have lesser priority may never be done. However, resolve to commit yourself to doing those activities that you value, and honour such commitments.

Develop a healthy attitude towards your body and your state of health

Undoubtedly you have heard it said that it is difficult to have mental health if you do not have physical health. Strictly speaking, this is not true. I know of individuals who are struck down by incapacitating illnesses, but this only seems to spur them on to greater mental resolve and ironically they may have become more mentally healthy than if they had not experienced the incapacitating disease. Yet it is also true that if you do not keep yourself in reasonable physical shape, then you may lose a sense of physical vitality, and in your lethargic state it will be harder for you to work steadily towards greater emotional well-being.

Realize, then, that you need to pay attention to your body and to your physical well-being. Don't be alarmed, I'm not about to lecture you on the evils of drink, tobacco and other substances which, if taken in excess, will do you harm. That would probably be the quickest way to get you to close this book. Nor am I about to give you a lecture on the importance of joining a health club and the necessity of taking frequent vigorous physical exercise. I am not about to do all this for two reasons. First of all, as a psychologist, I am not qualified to do so. Second, I do not want to preach to you. What I do want to stress, however, is the importance of paying *some* attention to your physical well-being and of realizing that if you do not, then it is likely that you will make yourself more vulnerable to physical deterioration later on and as a result your mental health will in all probability suffer.

I believe that here, as elsewhere, it is important to be flexible and to be moderate. So please do not become fanatical about any physical regime that you may choose to follow. Nor, I suggest, should you avoid exercise altogether. What I do advocate is that you consult your doctor and perhaps a nutritional specialist and ask them to outline a moderate plan of eating and exercise which will help you to keep your body in reasonable shape for the rest of your life.

I also advocate that you become aware of what I call your health vulnerabilities and to take whatever constructive or preventative measures expert medical and nutritional advice can give you. Often we live our lives as if we are immune from heart attacks, cancer and other life-threatening illnesses. It is only after we have experienced them that we choose to change our lifestyle. So again, without becoming fanatical, without turning to unproven fads and fancies that crop up every other year or so in popular magazines, give careful thought to what you can do to prevent, as far as you can, the development of such diseases. You cannot ward off all such illnesses, but an ounce of prevention may be worth more to you now than several pounds of invasive medical care later.

Learn to nurture yourself

By nurturing yourself, I mean treating yourself as you would somebody for whom you care. It is striking to note that we are often taught and shown models of how people nurture others, but we very rarely are taught or see healthy models of people who constructively and healthily nurture themselves. Let me give you a personal example of how I nurture myself, to give you an idea of what I mean. I personally find listening to Gregorian chant by monks immensely soothing. Once a day I set aside about 20 minutes for myself to do nothing but close my eyes and listen to one of my Gregorian monk chant recordings on my trusty iPod. Now, for you, doing the same might be anything but nurturing. I am not about to extol the virtues of Gregorian monk chants! What I do suggest is that you discover for yourself what activities or endeavours you can regularly participate in which you find soothing or nurturing. This might mean going for a regular massage or taking a walk in the woods. As I pointed out earlier in this book, human beings are extremely varied in their interests and, in this context, in what they experience as nurturing. So discover activities that you can do for yourself or with others, or that others can do for you, that are nurturing, and engage in these on a regular basis. You'll be surprised what impact it has on your emotional well-being.

Develop self-compassion

Recently, the concept of compassion has received much attention in the psychological literature. In particular, my friend and colleague Professor Paul Gilbert from the University of Derby has produced some innovative work, culminating in his book entitled *The Compassionate Mind* (Constable, 2010). He has argued that developing compassion acts as a protective mechanism against the development of depression. It also seems to be an important ingredient in the treatment of eating disorders.

Dr Kristin Neff from the University of Texas at Austin has contributed to our understanding of self-compassion by outlining its three main components, which you should try to implement in your own way.

- Self-kindness – being kind and understanding towards oneself in instances of pain or failure rather than being harshly self-critical. If you find this difficult, imagine yourself offering this ingredient to someone that you love and care for. Then apply it to yourself.
- Common humanity – perceiving one's experiences as part of the larger human experience rather than seeing them as separating and isolating. This is a particularly good counter to self-pity, where you see yourself as being singled out for unfair treatment by a cruel and uncaring world.
- Mindfulness* – holding painful thoughts and feelings in balanced awareness rather than over-identifying with them. This is a skill that I can't teach you here, but there are an increasing

---

* Since the first edition of this book came out in 1994, I would that say that the current interest in mindfulness is one of the most popular trends in the field of personal development. It is such an important topic that it warrants a book on its own, and as such I recommend *The Mindful Path to Self-Compassion* by Christopher K. Germer (Guilford Press, 2009).

number of courses being run on helping people to develop mindfulness and I suggest that, if you are interested in developing this skill, you search locally for one such course.

Strive to live up to your standards, values and ethics

Don't worry, I'm not about to give you a sermon! What I do want to encourage you to do is to consider carefully what your ethical standards, moral principles and values are, and to strive to live up to them. You are, of course, human and from time to time you may well fall short in doing this. If this happens, I recommend that you accept yourself and learn from the experience.

However, in my experience, those people who are happiest are those who live in reasonable accord with their standards, values and ethics. They have a sense that they are helping to create a world that they themselves would like to live in. They also seem more at peace with themselves than others who routinely go against what they hold dear in terms of ethics and values. If you have difficulty in discovering what your values are, I suggest that you consult a book called *Values Clarification*, written by Sidney B. Simon, Leland W. Howe and Howard Kirschenbaum (Warner Books, 1995).

Strive to be authentic

Let's face it, it is extraordinarily difficult to be genuine in this modern, complex, everyday world. Sociologists will tell you that you are being constantly encouraged to play roles, put on masks and hide your true feelings in the service of greater efficiency. Of course, it would be naive of me to say that you are not under such pressure. However, I do believe that you are still able to be reasonably authentic even in the face of these pressures.

There are two forms of authenticity that I want to discuss here. The first concerns being authentic with yourself. By this I mean that you are honest with yourself and do not try to hide your true feelings in a futile attempt to live up to an idealized but inhuman image (which is the quickest route to becoming estranged from your true feelings). Being honest with yourself is much easier, of course, if you have gone a reasonable way towards developing unconditional self-acceptance (USA), so you may wish to go back to the beginning of this step and reread the material on USA before proceeding. Assuming that you have gained a fair measure of USA, then, you need to pay attention to your feelings and true values, thoughts and beliefs. Try not to convince yourself that you are other than you are. People who are at peace with themselves acknowledge that they do have limitations and may, in a non-anxious but determined manner, address these limitations. However, people who are at odds with themselves either deny their faults and failings, project them on to others or try to change them in a desperate manner.

Being authentic with others is important, too, of course. Honestly disclosing your likes and dislikes to others, particularly at the beginning of a relationship, can save much heartache and much wasted time. How often have you put on your best – and often false – face to others because you believe that they could not accept you if you were truly honest with them? John Powell, a Jesuit priest, wrote a delightful book entitled *Why Am I Afraid To Tell You Who I Am?* (Zondervan, 1999). In it he shows that at the root of your fear of being authentic with others is, strange as it may seem, a lack of unconditional self-acceptance for your own weaknesses. Once you have achieved a fair measure of USA, you are likely to become more authentic with others. If they reject you, that is sad, but it is better that they reject you at the beginning of a relationship than much later, when you reveal your true feelings having kept them hidden for so long.

Please note that I am not urging you to be callous, crass and rude to people. I believe that you can tactfully disclose and communicate even strong negative feelings. I am not advocating an 'anything goes', 'let your feelings out', 'scream and yell' type of authenticity because this is healthy neither for you nor for those who are at the receiving end of such immature behaviour. What I am suggesting, and what I will say more about later in this book, is that you communicate your feelings honestly, but with care and tact. Here, as elsewhere, you need to be flexible in the expression of your authenticity!

Step 6

Allow yourself to experience healthy negative emotions

You may think it strange for me to include a section on experiencing negative emotions in a book on the promotion of mental health. However, I wish to dispel any ideas that you may have that people who are mentally healthy experience only positive feelings or react with calmness to life's adversities. Such a view of mental health is highly unrealistic. Indeed, if there are any individuals who experience only positive emotions, then either they have not encountered any adversities in their lives or they react to these adversities with inappropriate positive attitudes. Since your feelings stem from your beliefs, if you are able to feel positive about a negative event, this is because you hold an unrealistic positive belief about this event.

For example, let's suppose that you have entered a poetry competition and been told that you have been shortlisted for first prize. You are excited because you really wish to win this prize; it is very important to you. Then you receive a letter telling you that you did not win the competition. Isn't it unrealistic for you to believe, 'Good, I'm pleased that I didn't win the prize'? This is what you would have to believe in order to feel good about losing the competition. Now, you may have mixed positive and negative feelings about the event, and that is fine. For example, you may think, 'I'm sorry that I didn't win first prize, but I'm pleased to have had my poetry shortlisted.' However, the point to note is that your attitude, 'I'm sorry that I did not win the competition', would lead you to feel disappointed, which is a healthy, negative emotion. Although this feeling is negative in the sense that it feels unpleasant, it is healthy because it enables you to adjust to the negative event, process it and move on.

Now let's suppose that you are calm or indifferent about not winning first prize. Why would this also not be an example of good mental health? In Step 2, I said that as a human being you have a complex mixture of desires. You want certain things to happen and don't want other things to happen. When you receive bad news, such as not winning the poetry competition, this constitutes a frustration to your desire and thus it is healthy for you to have a negative feeling such as disappointment.

In order for you to have no feelings (i.e. calmness or indifference) about your failure to win the competition, you would have to hold a belief which would underpin this feeling or, more accurately, this lack of feeling. You would have to believe, in effect, that it doesn't matter to you whether or not you win the poetry competition. Now this sounds like a blatant piece of self-deception or an example of a defence mechanism that psychologists call 'denial'. When you hold an indifference belief you are acting like the fox in the story of the fox and the grapes. If you recall, the fox really wanted the grapes but could not reach them. Rather than healthily concluding that this was a disappointing experience and that maybe he needed to give some more thought to solving the problem of reaching the grapes, the fox concluded that he didn't want the grapes anyway since they were very likely to be sour.

I hope you can see now why I say that experiencing healthy negative emotions is a hallmark of mental health. If you only have positive emotions in life, this is likely to mean that you feel positively about negative life events, which is a highly unrealistic position. If you feel indifferent to certain things that you really want, then you are deceiving yourself and denying what is really important to you.

In the rest of this step, I will outline what I consider to be healthy negative emotions and show how these are based upon the rational beliefs discussed in Steps 2 to 5. Before I do so, I want to make an important point about terminology. Unfortunately, in the English language we do not have agreed terms for either unhealthy negative emotions or healthy negative emotions. The terms I use here are the ones most frequently used in Rational Emotive Behaviour Therapy (REBT), but what is more important is that you employ terms that are meaningful to you. As you do so, make sure you use words that keenly differentiate a healthy negative emotion from an unhealthy negative emotion.

In what follows, I will compare these with their unhealthy negative counterparts, which are based on the irrational beliefs also discussed in those steps. So, reread those sections for a detailed discussion of the rational and irrational beliefs that I have already covered. Here, I will give you a very brief reminder before we continue.

It is my view that the healthy negative emotions that I am about to consider stem from one or more of the following rational beliefs:

- a flexible belief with respect to your desires;
- a non-awfulizing belief coupled with an acceptance of reality;
- a discomfort tolerance belief;
- an unconditional acceptance belief about self, others and the world.

Unhealthy negative emotions stem from one or more of the following beliefs:

- a rigid belief with respect to your desires;
- an awfulizing belief which leads you to get things out of proportion;
- a discomfort intolerance belief;
- a depreciation belief about self, others and the world.

Concern (the healthy alternative to anxiety)

When you are faced with a threat to your safety, well-being, comfort or view of yourself, then it is healthy to be concerned about this threat. Hiding your head in the sand and pretending that the threat does not exist will not help you to confront and deal with it, nor will rushing around like a headless chicken in an anxious frame of mind.

Concern stems from the following set of beliefs. 'If a threat exists, all the conditions are unfortunately in place for it to exist. It would be nice if it did not exist, but there is no law of the universe which states that it must not exist. Furthermore, it is bad that the threat exists, but not awful. I am able to put up with the situation and deal with the threat if and when it occurs, and if it does, I can still unconditionally accept myself, others and the world under such circumstances.'

Anxiety is the unhealthy counterpart to concern in the face of threat. When you feel anxious about a threat, you insist that it must not occur, that it would be horrible if it did, that you cannot stand it and that if the threat is to your view of yourself, and it was to materialize, it would prove that you were worthless. Experiencing concern about a threat is healthy because:

- it helps you to acknowledge that the threat exists;
- it enables you to think clearly and be motivated to deal with the threat constructively if it materializes, or to make alternative self-enhancing plans if the threat cannot be nullified.

In addition, if you experience concern rather than anxiety, you are far less likely to overestimate the degree of the threat or danger. I have carried out research studies which show that this last point is the case.

In one of the studies, I asked one group of subjects to hold a set of rational but realistically negative beliefs towards spiders. This group was told to keep in mind the following: 'I would prefer not to see a spider, but if I do it would be unfortunate but not terrible. It is uncomfortable seeing a spider but not unbearable.' The second group was asked to hold a set of irrational beliefs towards spiders. They were asked to keep in mind the following: 'I must not see a spider. If I were to see one it would be horrible and unbearable.' Both these groups were asked to imagine that they were going into a room where there was at least one spider; they were asked a number of questions concerning the number of spiders that were likely to be in the room, their size and the direction of their movement.

It will not surprise you to learn that, compared to the group who were asked to hold a set of rational beliefs, the group who were asked to hold a set of irrational beliefs towards spiders guessed that there would be more spiders, that such spiders would be larger, and that the spiders would be more likely to be moving towards them. This experiment shows that if you hold an anxiety-related set of irrational beliefs, you overestimate the degree of threat in your environment. You also tend to underestimate your ability to cope with the threat. However, if you experience unanxious concern, you neither overestimate the threat nor underestimate your ability to cope with it.

For more information on how to feel concerned rather than anxious in the face of adversity, see my book for Sheldon Press entitled *Overcoming Anxiety* (2000).

Sadness (as opposed to depression)

Whenever you have lost something that is important to you, failed at something important or experienced an undeserved plight, it is healthy for you to feel sad about the loss/failure/undeserved plight. To shrug off these adversities as if they are of no or little importance to you will not help you to integrate such experiences, recharge your batteries and move on with your life. However, if you feel depressed about the loss/failure/undeserved plight, this is not healthy because depression discourages you from taking action and leads you to be emotionally stuck.

Sadness about a loss, failure or undeserved plight stems from the following set of rational beliefs: 'It is undesirable for the loss/failure/undeserved plight to have occurred but there is no law of the universe that states that it absolutely shouldn't have happened. If it happened, it happened. It is bad that the loss/failure/undeserved plight occurred, but not terrible. It is bearable and (if appropriate) does not reflect on my worth as a person.'

However, if you are depressed about the loss/failure/undeserved plight, it is likely that you believe that this adversity absolutely should not have happened, that it is unbearable and (if relevant) proves something worthless about you.

When you are sad, but not depressed, about a loss/failure/undeserved plight, you do not feel hopeless about the future. You recognize that experiencing such adversities is a part of the complex business of living and that it is important to integrate them into a wider view of the world. However, when you are depressed, you tend to feel hopeless about the future. If you feel hopeless about the future you will tend to contemplate suicide. Life loses its meaning because you do not accept that such losses/failures/undeserved plights should occur, if the conditions exist for them to occur.

Sadness helps you to grieve and move on and encourages you to take constructive action. Depression tends either to inhibit the grieving process or to extend it. Also, when you are depressed, you will not feel like taking any action at all and that which you do take is unlikely to be constructive. So, by all means strive to feel sad about your losses, failures and undeserved plights, but try to minimize feelings of depression by identifying and challenging the irrational beliefs that underpin this unconstructive, negative emotion.

For more information concerning how to feel sad rather than depressed in the face of adversity, see my book for Sheldon Press entitled *Overcoming Depression* (2003), which I wrote with Sarah Opie.

Healthy anger (as opposed to unhealthy anger)

When another person frustrates you, threatens your view of yourself or breaks one of your important personal rules, it is unhealthy for you to turn the other cheek, to offer the person loving kindness or to be indifferent towards his or her behaviour. Rather, in my view, when these undesirable events happen it is constructive for you to be healthily angry about such eventualities. If one of your colleagues at work has tried to stab you in the back by spreading a false rumour about you, do you really think it is constructive to turn the other cheek and feel nothing? No, I think it is very healthy for you to feel anger at what this person has done and to try to redeem the situation constructively. However, there are two types of anger, healthy anger and unhealthy anger, and only the first is constructive.

When you are healthily angry, you believe:

- 'It would be preferable for such frustrations, etc., not to occur, but that does not mean that they must not occur';
- 'It is quite unfortunate when they occur, but not terrible';
- 'It is uncomfortable, but not intolerable';

- 'The other person who frustrates me is a person who has acted in a bad manner but is not a bad person.'*

Unhealthy anger, however, which is at the root of much interpersonal conflict and tends to ruin rather than improve relations, tends to stem from a demanding philosophy where you believe:

- 'The other person absolutely must not break my rules or frustrate me';
- 'It is terrible that he or she did';
- 'The situation is unbearable';
- 'The other person is a thoroughgoing blackguard for acting in such a bad manner.'

If you are unhealthily angry and you choose to express it, you will raise your blood pressure. You will also get into additional trouble with the other person because she (in this case) will experience you as damning her rather than just disliking her behaviour. Even if you manage to intimidate the other person, you will encourage her in future to exact revenge on you. If you don't express your unhealthy anger, you are also in trouble because it is likely that you will develop a whole host of psychosomatic symptoms. You may attempt to get back at the other person through passive-aggressive means and you will generally be ill at ease with yourself and the world.

However, if you are healthily angry, you are more likely to try to change the situation constructively by engaging the other person in a dialogue where you tell her honestly how you feel about her behaviour, while indicating strongly that you are not damning her. In fact, you accept her unconditionally as a fallible individual and indicate a wish to resolve the issue and resume good relationships.

So, whenever somebody does something that breaks your rules, threatens your view of yourself or frustrates you in the pursuit of your desires, don't turn the other cheek or feel indifferent: be healthily angry and try to deal with the situation constructively.

---

* The points that I put forward in discussing unconditional self-acceptance beliefs in Step 5 also hold for unconditional other-acceptance.

For more information concerning how to feel healthy anger rather than unhealthy anger in the face of adversity, see my book for Sheldon Press entitled *Overcoming Anger: When anger helps and when it hurts* (1996).

Remorse (as opposed to guilt)

Have you ever (a) failed to live up to a moral code or ethical principle, (b) acted in a way that conflicts with your moral values or (c) hurt someone's feelings? Most, if not all, of us have, and most people believe it is healthy to feel guilty about such lapses from ethical behaviour. If you define guilt carefully and distinguish it keenly from its healthy counterpart – constructive remorse – I think you will see that guilt is not a constructive, healthy response to situations where you 'fall from grace'. Guilt stems from the following philosophy: 'I absolutely must not break my moral code, fail to live up to this code or hurt someone's feelings. If I do so it is terrible, I cannot stand the situation and I am a bad, wicked sinner for so doing.' Holding this set of irrational beliefs will, in fact, encourage you to act badly in the future, because if it is true that you are a bad, wicked person, how do bad, wicked people act other than badly and wickedly?

Now, before you assume that I am condoning immoral behaviour, etc., let me make it quite clear that I am not. Whenever you break or fail to live up to your moral code or hurt someone's feelings, I want you to feel remorseful (but not guilty) about this. If you do, you will hold the following beliefs:

- 'I acted badly* and I wish that I hadn't. However, there is no law in the universe which states that I must not act badly.'
- 'This situation is bad and calls for me to reflect on what I've done. However, it is not terrible.'
- 'It is uncomfortable to act against my moral code, but it's not unbearable.'

---

* This includes breaking your moral code, failing to live up to said code or hurting someone's feelings.

- 'I am a fallible human being who did a bad thing, but I am not a blackguard.'

I believe that these rational beliefs, which are at the root of constructive remorse, will encourage you to reflect on your behaviour and increase the chance that you will learn from your mistakes. When you experience self-blaming guilt, you will either be so consumed with your own wickedness that you won't learn from your errors or you will be motivated to deny responsibility for your behaviour.

So, recognize that, as a fallible human being, you will at times fail to live up to your ethical standards. Accept yourself as a fallible human being and allow yourself to feel remorseful, learn from your errors and make appropriate amends for your behaviour. Desist from damning yourself as an unworthy, evil sinner since this will only encourage you to act badly in the future, either because that's what evil people do or because guilt interferes with your ability to learn from your mistakes.

For more information concerning how to feel remorse rather than guilt in the face of adversity, see my book for Sheldon Press entitled *Coping with Guilt* (2013).

Disappointment (as opposed to shame)

People often confuse guilt with shame. While they both involve you depreciating yourself, these emotions are about different things and the content of your self-depreciation is different. As I showed you above, when you feel guilty, you think that you have broken or failed to live up to your moral code or you think that you have hurt someone's feelings and you consider yourself bad for your moral lapses. As we have seen, the healthy alternative to guilt is remorse, where you accept yourself unconditionally while taking full responsibility for your behaviour.

By contrast, you feel shame when:

- you think that you have fallen short of your ideal, where your behaviour has shown your reference group in a bad light and/or others look down on you, shun you or are disgusted with your behaviour;

- you demand that one or more of the above absolutely should not have happened and because it did you are defective, disgusting or diminished as a person.

The healthy alternative to shame is disappointment. You experience disappointment when you again think that:

- you have fallen short of your ideal, where your behaviour has shown your reference group in a bad light and/or others look down on you, shun you or are disgusted with your behaviour.

However, this time you hold a set of rational beliefs about these inferences, namely:

- You prefer that one or more of the above had not happened, but you do not demand that they absolutely should not have happened. If it has happened, you accept yourself unconditionally as a complex, fallible human being who is neither defective, disgusting nor diminished as a person.

When you experience disappointment rather than shame, you are more likely to stay in the situation and face your accusers with your head held high rather than withdraw from them or avoid their gaze. When disappointed, you are also more likely to take a compassionate and understanding view of your behaviour and resolve to learn from any mistakes you have made. By contrast, when you feel ashamed, you cannot even bear to think of what you have done and, as a result, you won't learn anything from the situation.

For more information concerning how to feel disappointment rather than shame in the face of adversity, see my book for Sheldon Press entitled *Overcoming Shame* (1997).

Sorrow (as opposed to hurt and self-pity)

As I showed in my book *The Incredible Sulk* (Sheldon Press, 1992), a large part of the sulking experience is hurt and self-pity. When you are experiencing hurt and self-pity, you will tend to hold the following beliefs about the unfair or undeserving way you have been treated:

- 'Because I don't deserve unfair treatment it absolutely must not happen.'
- 'Because I have been treated unfairly it is terrible and the world is a rotten place for allowing this to happen to such an undeserving creature as me.'

When you feel hurt and self-pity, does this help you to deal constructively with the unfairness or not? My clinical experience indicates that people who experience hurt and self-pity tend to withdraw from constructive communication rather than engage in it. They either sulk, loudly or quietly, or engage others in an endless 'ain't it awful' type of conversation. In addition, they may try to elicit sympathy and pity from their nearest and dearest, which if they are successful only serves to strengthen their own self-pitying attitude.

What, then, is the constructive alternative to hurt and self-pity? The answer is sorrow; it is healthy to feel sorrowful if you have been treated unfairly and in a way that you believe you do not deserve. There is an important distinction between sorrow and self-pity. In self-pity you believe that you are a poor creature for receiving such treatment, whereas if you are sorrowful, but not self-pitying, you believe that you are a person who is in a poor situation but who is not to be pitied as a person. Furthermore, if you are in a sorrowful, but not self-pitying, frame of mind, you are likely to believe:

- 'While it is undesirable to be treated in an unfair, undeserving manner, there is no law of the universe that says that fairness and deservingness must exist';
- 'If the unfairness exists, then it is bad but not terrible';
- 'It is a situation that I can stand and therefore can try to correct';
- 'The world is hardly a rotten place but is a complex environment in which bad and good things happen; it is a place where, if I think about it, I experience certain unfairnesses which are in my favour.'

This last point is important. It is likely that most of you reading this book are in good health, have all your mental faculties and all your limbs intact. Isn't this situation unfair to those people who are in poor health, who have lost limbs or who do not have all their mental faculties intact? When we focus on unfairness in our favour it is unlikely that we insist that these must not exist! So, when you are self-pitying, you are over-focused on unfairness which is against you and you neglect or edit out completely unfairness in your favour.

For more information concerning how to feel sorrow rather than hurt in the face of adversity, see my book for Sheldon Press entitled *Overcoming Hurt* (2007).

Healthy jealousy (as opposed to unhealthy jealousy)

When you experience healthy jealousy there is clear evidence that you are facing a threat to your relationship (e.g. with your partner) and you hold the following set of rational beliefs about this threat:

- 'I don't want this threat to exist, but it does not mean that it must not do so.'
- 'It's unfortunate that this threat exists, but it's not terrible.'
- 'It's hard to tolerate the existence of this threat, but I can do so and it's worth tolerating.'
- 'This threat does not impact on my self-esteem. I'm the same fallible human being whether or not the threat exists.'

This set of rational beliefs will help you to engage your partner in a productive discussion of the meaning of the threat for his or her feelings for you and the other person, and of the implications for your relationship with your partner.

By contrast, when you feel unhealthily jealous, you hold the following set of rational beliefs:

- 'This threat must not exist.'
- 'It's awful that it does.'
- 'I can't bear that the threat exists.'
- 'This threat proves that I am less worthy than my rival.'

Unhealthy jealousy does not facilitate a productive discussion between you and your partner. Rather, it leads to behaviour that will threaten your relationship more seriously than any rival. Thus, when you are unhealthily jealous you tend to sulk, become aggressive, cross-examine your partner, check on his or her whereabouts and set traps for him or her. You tend not to do any of these when you are healthily jealous.

Finally, when you hold the irrational beliefs that underpin unhealthy jealousy, you will tend to interpret the existence of threats to your relationship when little or no evidence is present for the existence of such a threat. Again, you tend not to do this when you hold the rational beliefs that underpin healthy jealousy.

For more information concerning how to feel healthy jealousy rather than unhealthy jealousy in the face of adversity, see my book for Sheldon Press entitled *Overcoming Jealousy* (1998).

Healthy envy (as opposed to unhealthy envy)

You tend to experience envy (whether healthy or unhealthy) when another person has something that you prize but do not have. Healthy envy, once again, is based on a set of rational beliefs such as:

- 'I would like to have what the other has, but I don't need to have it.'
- 'It's bad to be deprived in this way, but it is certainly not terrible.'
- 'I can bear this deprivation, although it is difficult to put up with. However, it is worth it to me to do so.'
- 'I am the same person whether or not I have what the other person has.'

This set of rational beliefs will lead you to pursue the prized 'object' only if you really want it and can get pleasure or use out of it. In unhealthy envy, by contrast, you pursue the 'object' whether or not you really want it and will use it. In healthy envy, you do not experience any urge to deprive the other person of the prized object or spoil it for him or her, while in unhealthy envy you do have these urges and will sometimes act on them.

Unhealthy envy, for the record, is based on the following set of irrational beliefs:

- 'I must have what the other has.'
- 'It's awful to be deprived.'
- 'I can't bear the deprivation.'
- 'This deprivation means that I am less worthy than I would be if I had what I prize and that I am less worthy than the other person is.'

For more information concerning how to feel healthy envy rather than unhealthy envy in the face of adversity, see my book for Sheldon Press entitled *Coping with Envy* (2010).

Conclusion

In conclusion, I want to reiterate that when adversities occur in your life, it is not healthy to put on a brave face and look only for the good in the experience. It is also not healthy to adopt an attitude of indifference and unconcern. Rather, when you encounter adversity in your life it is constructive for you to be concerned, sad, healthily angry, remorseful, disappointed, sorrowful, healthily jealous or healthily envious. Don't try to change these feelings. Allow yourself to experience them, because they will help you to deal with the situation constructively and to make a healthy adjustment, if indeed you cannot change these negative events. However, if you experience anxiety, depression, unhealthy anger, guilt, shame, hurt or self-pity, unhealthy jealousy or unhealthy envy, look for the irrational beliefs that underpin such emotions, challenge and change them (see Step 10) and work towards experiencing healthy, negative feelings instead.

Step 7

Think critically and creatively

In my dealings with people who are, in my opinion, mentally healthy, I have been struck by their ability to think critically and creatively. Such people do not accept what they are told without thinking it through for themselves. This ability to think for themselves enables them to resist the power of advertising and the false claims of self-styled experts. Thus, people who think for themselves tend not to be naive and gullible. Rather, they listen carefully to what they are told, consider the motives of those who are talking to them and form their own judgements.

Think scientifically

A major aspect of the ability to think critically is the adoption of the scientific method. Scientific thinking is the hallmark of healthy scepticism. When you think scientifically, you advance a hypothesis which you then test out by looking for evidence which either supports or contradicts your hypothesis. In order to do this you need a degree of objectivity. It is perhaps a paradox when I say that many scientists are not good scientific thinkers. This is because they are over-invested in the results of their experiments, which they hope will confirm their favourite hypothesis. Scientific literature is full of examples where scientists have either fraudulently altered the results of their experiments to confirm their favourite hypothesis, or have failed to institute proper scientific controls with the consequence that the results are biased towards supporting their favourite hypothesis. In order to think scientifically, therefore, it is important that you do not become over-invested in proving to yourself that your hypotheses are true. This involves taking into account what you want to happen so that you minimize the biasing effect of your desires. This is difficult, as Nassim Nicholas Taleb has noted in his excellent book of philosophical and practical aphorisms entitled *The Bed of Procrustes* (Random House, 2011). In particular, he says: 'The person you are the most afraid to contradict is yourself' (p. 3).

Let's suppose, for example, that you have been told that you have contracted a debilitating but non-life-threatening disease. You are also told that there is no medication that you can take that will help you. Let's suppose that, two weeks after you are told this, you read in a newspaper that some self-styled expert has discovered a remedy that you can take to minimize the effects of this disease on your life. How can you apply critical scientific thinking to this situation? First of all, it would be important for you to find out a lot more, both about the advertised remedy, in particular its ingredients, and also about the qualifications of the self-styled expert. Many people have failed to make such sensible checks and have had their hopes cruelly raised and dashed by unscrupulous individuals whose sole motivation is to make money. Having gathered as much information as you can about the ingredients of the remedy and the qualifications of the so-called expert, show this information to people who *are* recognized authorities in the field. Listen carefully to these authorities, but watch out for any axes that they have to grind. I say this because many respected medical authorities are dogmatically opposed to anything that smacks of what is known as alternative medicine.

Now, analyse all the information you have collected and then make a decision. If you decide to take the remedy, do so for a limited period and note carefully the effects on your condition. Then stop taking the remedy and note the effects of this withdrawal on your symptoms. Start taking the solution again and note carefully what changes, if any, you experience in your symptoms as a consequence. If, as a result of approaching this problem scientifically, you discover that you have in fact gained benefit from the remedy, then by all means continue to take it. If, however, it seems as if there is no effect over and above an initial improvement in your symptoms – which would probably be due to your understandable desire for it to work – then there is really no point in continuing to take it. Approaching this and other problems in a systematic and scientific manner will enable you to feel more in control of the decisions that you make, and will make you far less prey to the fads and magical solutions that are constantly on offer in this entrepreneurial world.

Minimize the effects of poisonous pedagogy

When you are taught various things about yourself, other people and the world by significant others, like parents, teachers and ministers, which are unduly negative and, if you believe them, self-defeating, this is poisonous pedagogy.

You may have grown up hearing one or both of your parents, for example, give you the following messages:

- 'You're just like your father, good for nothing.'
- 'People aren't to be trusted. Stick to the family, they'll look after you.' (Here the implication is that other people will seek to take advantage of you.)
- 'All men are only after one thing.'
- 'Women just want to hook you and then bleed you dry.'

If you are repeatedly exposed to such poisonous teachings at a time when you are impressionable and find it difficult to think for yourself, it is no surprise that you may come to believe such unwarranted views of the world. If you believe them then they will have a decided influence on how you feel and how you act in the world. Thus, if you believe that all women are out to entrap you, you may well only develop brief and superficial relationships with females, avoiding the possibility of establishing any lasting relationships with them. Furthermore, if you believe that people outside your family are only out to take advantage of you, this will affect the degree to which you disclose your thoughts, feelings and attitudes to them.

You may find it a very useful exercise to sit down and ask yourself, 'What were the basic messages that I learned about myself, other people and the world from significant others in my life?' Take a piece of paper and write down who these significant others were and just what they taught you about yourself, other people and the world in general. The more specific you are, the more you will be able to stand back and re-evaluate these messages.

When you do come to re-evaluate these messages, bear the following in mind. First, it is almost certain that any statement which
has the word 'all' in it is an unwarranted overgeneralization (e.g.
'All men are only after one thing'). This means that it may have a
kernel of truth to it; for example, some men may only be after one
thing, but it is hardly likely that *all* men are *only* after one thing.

Second, ask yourself whether a particular message says more
about yourself, other people or the world in general, or more about
the person who taught you this way of looking at yourself, others
and the world. Considering what you know about the source of
the message, could what that person taught you have been heavily
influenced by his or her own attitudes and perhaps by what he or
she was taught by significant others in his or her own past? Family
therapists have pointed out that statements about people and the
world in general may be handed down from generation to generation. The reason for this is that each generation accepts these messages uncritically.

Third, when you start to re-evaluate the poisonous messages
from your past, bear in mind you can always find some evidence
to support these messages. Thus, if you think about your dealings
with people outside your family, you may well be able to identify
situations when, indeed, you were taken advantage of. However,
just because you may find such evidence doesn't mean that the
overgeneralized message is true. In addition, you may be operating
according to a self-fulfilling prophecy. A self-fulfilling prophecy
occurs when, by your own actions, you bring about an outcome
that supports the belief that you held in the first place. Thus, if you
believe that nobody outside the family is to be trusted, you may
act naively towards a stranger who takes advantage of you. Instead
of concluding that this is more evidence that people outside your
family are not to be trusted, you need to consider your own role
in this episode.

What I am saying here is that once you have uncritically accepted
poisonous messages from your past, you may unwittingly seek out
experiences which confirm these views because, like many people,
you prefer familiarity to unfamiliarity. Take, for example, a situation where you meet somebody who seems trustworthy. Remember your basic position: people outside the family are not to be

trusted. As a result, the more you get to know this person the more unfamiliar your experience will be. Given the choice between surrendering a poisonous but familiar message and realizing that perhaps your parents were wrong and that people outside the family can be trusted, on the one hand, and maintaining your belief in that message and bringing about an untrustworthy response from this other person, on the other, you may well do the latter. Thus, you may unwittingly take advantage of this other person, who may respond in kind. Forgetting or even not realizing your own actions and their likely impact, you may just focus on the other person's untrustworthy response and conclude that your parents were right all along: other people outside the family are not to be trusted.

You need to realize that if you are to change such poisonous messages about yourself, other people and the world, you will be entering into the realm of the unfamiliar. As such you will be tempted to doctor your experiences to support the poisonous message rather than stay with the unfamiliarity so that you can re-evaluate the message. What you need, then, is a high degree of tolerance for discomfort and unfamiliarity if you are to stay with the experiences which fail to confirm the poisonous pedagogy (see Step 4).

Minimize your distorted thinking

The famous American psychiatrist Aaron T. Beck, founder of Cognitive Therapy, has argued that when people are in emotional distress, they frequently show distortions in the way that they think about themselves, other people and the world. It is my view that these distortions often stem from the four unhealthy beliefs discussed in Steps 2 to 5. Thus, if you hold rigid beliefs, awfulizing beliefs, discomfort intolerance beliefs and depreciation beliefs about self, others and the world, your thinking about the events in your life will show very many distortions. It follows that one of the major ways of taking the distortions out of your thinking is to identify and change the above-listed four irrational beliefs. I will show you how to do this in Step 10. Thus, if you hold flexible beliefs about your desires and non-awfulizing beliefs about life's adversities, if you raise your discomfort tolerance and operate from a position of unconditional acceptance of self, others and the world, you will go a long way towards thinking clearly and accurately about the events in your life.

After you have done this, you will be in a better position both emotionally and objectively to identify and correct any distortions that remain in your thinking. What are some of the major thinking distortions that impede mental health? Below, I list some of the major ones.

Black-and-white thinking

Here, you use only two categories in your attempt to make sense of an experience. In black-and-white thinking there are literally no shades of grey (e.g. 'Either I do perfectly well or I have failed miserably'). To change black-and-white thinking you need to appreciate that things are rarely black and white and that there are many different shades of grey in your experiences. Thus, you may have achieved a mark of 80 per cent, and while this does not constitute a perfect performance it hardly represents a total failure. You may wish to acknowledge the disappointment of not scoring 100 per cent on the test, but it is important also to acknowledge what you have achieved.

Jumping to unwarranted conclusions

Here, an event happens and you make an unwarranted negative conclusion from that event. David Burns, the author of the classic Cognitive Therapy self-help book *Feeling Good: The new mood therapy* (Avon Books, 1999), has identified two major forms of conclusion-jumping: mind-reading and fortune-telling.

Mind-reading

Here, you think you know what another person is thinking, based on little or no supporting data. An example of this may be when you go to a party and you conclude that other people must be thinking you are boring, despite the fact that those very people were listening attentively to what you were saying.

Fortune-telling

Here, you make a prediction about the future without having any definitive evidence that this event will happen. For example, you tell yourself that you will fail to be offered the job at an interview that you will be attending that afternoon.

Focusing on the negative and disqualifying the positive

In this distortion, you literally focus on the negative aspects of any experience and edit out, deny or disqualify any positive features of that experience. Thus, a teacher hands you back your essay on which she has made some very praiseworthy comments. In addition, she has pointed out two or three places where improvement is necessary. Using this distortion you completely disqualify the positive aspects of the praise, saying to yourself that the teacher is only trying to boost your ego, and you focus exclusively on the negative and use this as evidence to begin to feel depressed.

Emotional and cognitive reasoning

In these distortions, it is your view that because you feel a certain way or think a certain way, these constitute accurate evidence about reality. Thus you might say, 'Because I *feel* like a failure this proves that I really *am* a failure', or you may think, 'I won't give a good performance at the poetry reading tonight because I *think* that it will go poorly.' While your feelings and thoughts can be accurate statements about reality, to assume that this is necessarily so without reflecting critically on your feeling and thinking statements is to live your life on the assumption that the world is inevitably the way you feel and think it is. Doing so means that you will be unduly influenced in the way you view the world by your feeling and thinking prejudices.

Personalization

When you personalize an event, you either assume that you are the centre of the experience or that you are responsible for the experience. Many years ago a friend and I were laughing and joking about something to do with our favourite football team, and as we were doing so we passed a busker. The busker shouted after us, 'What's funny about my music?' This was a clear case of personalization in that the busker thought that our laughter was directed at him, whereas up to that point we had been unaware of his very existence.

In the other form of personalization, you assume that you are responsible for events that are really the responsibility of other people. If you hold this distortion you probably experience a lot of guilt in your life. Thus, you might conclude that you are responsible for your daughter's failure in her mathematics exam because you did not monitor her work habits. In this example, you are taking too much responsibility for this event and not giving enough responsibility to your daughter for failing to do the work necessary to pass the exam.

How to correct thinking distortions

An important first step in correcting a thinking distortion is to identify it properly. Thus, you need to familiarize yourself with the different types of distortions discussed in this section so that you can tell if you are thinking clearly or distortedly.

Second, having identified a distortion, the next step is to stand back and ask for evidence that both supports and contradicts your way of thinking. It is very important to carry out both of these steps, because if you just look for evidence to confirm your hypothesis, you may well find one or two features of the situation that support it. However, if you also look for evidence to contradict the hypothesis, you may find that such evidence outweighs the supportive evidence.

Third, you need to ask yourself, 'What alternative ways of viewing the same situation are there?' Here, you need to brainstorm and write down all the possible alternative views that you can think of. Then, ask yourself how somebody else who is not involved in this situation would view it. Would that person view it in the same way you did or would his or her view be more in line with one or more of the alternative views that you have developed?

Fourth, look for evidence to support these alternative ways of viewing the situation as well as for evidence that may go against these alternatives.

The final step is to stand back and choose the alternative which seems the most plausible, given all the steps you have taken so far and all the information you have gathered. While you can rarely see reality exactly as it is, you can choose the best way of viewing the experience, which is the way that has the most evidence to support it. If you wish to look further into the area of thinking distortions and how to correct them, read *Feeling Good: The new mood therapy* by David Burns (Avon Books, 1999).

I want to reiterate a point that I made earlier in this step. The best way to correct thinking distortions is first to challenge the irrational beliefs discussed in Steps 2 to 5 of this book. Thus, first identify and challenge your rigid beliefs, your awfulizing beliefs, your discomfort intolerance beliefs and your depreciation beliefs about self, others and the world. I will show you how to do this in Step 10. You will then be in a more realistic frame of mind to identify and correct any thinking distortions that still remain in the way that you view events.

Develop a problem-solving attitude

Problem-solving is a valuable, comprehensive method which you use in your daily life to solve both practical and emotional problems. The purpose of problem-solving is to encourage you to assume responsibility for your problems (see Step 1) and to develop a method of dealing with them which emphasizes discovering alternative and possibly more successful ways of coping with the problem.

There are nine stages in the problem-solving sequence:

1 Identify the problem as clearly and as unambiguously as you can.
2 Set realistic, achievable, specific goals. These may be divided into short-term and long-term goals.
3 List all the possible ways of solving the problem, no matter how bizarre some may sound. This is known as brainstorming alternatives.
4 List the pros and cons of each alternative.
5 Choose from your list the best alternative.
6 Plan how to implement this alternative, deciding on the steps you need to take to do this. Making a written step-by-step plan at this point is particularly useful.
7 Make a commitment to implement your chosen solution, specifying when, where and how you are going to do it.

8 After you have implemented your chosen solution, sit down and review what progress you have made towards your goal. At this point, decide what further steps you need to take in order to achieve your objective.

9 Evaluate the outcome of your chosen solution and decide whether other courses of action are necessary.

The best time to carry out a problem-solving procedure, like the one discussed above, is when you are not under the influence of any unhealthy negative emotions that you have about the problem at hand. It is difficult to see clearly when you are emotionally disturbed about a situation, and thinking clearly is the very thing that you need to do when you are employing the problem-solving procedure. So, first get yourself into a healthy frame of mind by challenging and changing your irrational beliefs (see Step 10) and then use the nine problem-solving stages outlined above.

Improve your decision-making

Many people find making decisions difficult. It is important to distinguish between difficulties in making decisions because of lack of information, and indecisiveness. Indecisiveness stems from one or more of a number of self-defeating beliefs which need to be identified and challenged before sensible decision-making procedures are used.

Indecisiveness may occur when you believe the following:

'I must be sure that I will make the right decision' While such a state of certainty would be nice, it is not a necessary precondition for decision-making. Indeed, it is impossible to know in advance that you are making the right decision. All you can do is gain the necessary information, make a decision and evaluate later whether it turns out to be right or wrong. In addition, it is impossible to be certain about anything, let alone the outcome of your decisions.

'I must be comfortable when I make decisions' While being comfortable may be desirable it is also not a necessary precondition for making a decision. Indeed, apart from decisions which are quite clear-cut, where there are only advantages to one course of action

and disadvantages to another course of action, most decisions involve choosing between alternatives that have both advantages and disadvantages. As such, making a decision invariably involves you putting up with a degree of discomfort since you are giving up some advantages of the non-preferred decision when you opt for the preferred decision.

'I must make the right decision, and if I don't, this proves that I am stupid and inadequate' Obviously, making the right decision is preferable – but necessary? Hardly! Even if you make what turns out to be a wrong decision, this is scarcely evidence of you being an inadequate person. It may be evidence that you have not taken enough time or collected enough information before making the decision. Or it may be evidence that certain factors that you could not possibly have known about come into play. If you were an inadequate person, every decision and, in fact, everything that you could ever do in life would be inadequate, which is an arrant overgeneralization.

Once you have identified, challenged and changed such self-defeating beliefs you are in a position to utilize the cost–benefit analysis procedure, which is designed to help you make effective decisions (see Figures 7.1 and 7.2 overleaf).

There are six steps that you need to take when you undertake a cost–benefit analysis. I will describe the six steps with reference to choosing between two options, but you can use this procedure with more than two options. You will find it helpful to have a notebook handy.

1 Clearly describe the two options (A and B) that you need to choose between. In your notebook, copy out the cost–benefit analysis form and write the options at the top of each section.
2 Take one of the options (e.g. option A) and focus on the advantages and benefits of choosing this option, in both the short term and the long term, for yourself and for other people.
3 Write down the corresponding disadvantages and costs of choosing this option, again in the short term and the long term, for yourself and for others.
4 Repeat the advantages and disadvantages analysis for the other option (B).

Advantages/costs of Option A

SHORT TERM

For yourself

1 _____
2 _____
3 _____
4 _____
5 _____
6 _____

For other people

1 _____
2 _____
3 _____
4 _____
5 _____
6 _____

LONG TERM

For yourself

1 _____
2 _____
3 _____
4 _____
5 _____
6 _____

For other people

1 _____
2 _____
3 _____
4 _____
5 _____
6 _____

Disadvantages/costs of Option A

SHORT TERM

For yourself

1 _____
2 _____
3 _____
4 _____
5 _____
6 _____

For other people

1 _____
2 _____
3 _____
4 _____
5 _____
6 _____

LONG TERM

For yourself

1 _____
2 _____
3 _____
4 _____
5 _____
6 _____

For other people

1 _____
2 _____
3 _____
4 _____
5 _____
6 _____

Figure 7.1 Cost–benefit analysis, Option A

Advantages/costs of Option B

SHORT TERM

For yourself

1 _____
2 _____
3 _____
4 _____
5 _____
6 _____

For other people

1 _____
2 _____
3 _____
4 _____
5 _____
6 _____

LONG TERM

For yourself

1 _____
2 _____
3 _____
4 _____
5 _____
6 _____

For other people

1 _____
2 _____
3 _____
4 _____
5 _____
6 _____

Disadvantages/costs of Option B

SHORT TERM

For yourself

1 _____
2 _____
3 _____
4 _____
5 _____
6 _____

For other people

1 _____
2 _____
3 _____
4 _____
5 _____
6 _____

LONG TERM

For yourself

1 _____
2 _____
3 _____
4 _____
5 _____
6 _____

For other people

1 _____
2 _____
3 _____
4 _____
5 _____
6 _____

Figure 7.2 Cost–benefit analysis, Option B

5 Go away for an hour or so and clear your head before coming back to your notebook and reviewing what you have written. Read your responses on each page and ask yourself the following question: on balance, and taking everything into account, is it better that I choose option A or option B?

6 Make your decision without any further debate. Even if it is very close, go for the option which overall has the slight edge. Make a commitment to implement it, and then implement it. Even if you make a wrong decision, you will often be happier in the long term than if you postpone, prevaricate and continue an indecisive approach to decision-making.

Develop your creativity

Being creative involves a process called divergent thinking. This involves taking risks with your thinking in ways that may defy logic, appear absurd and seem foolish to other people. As such, creative thinking frequently involves the temporary suspension of critical thinking to enable new ideas to develop, new associations to form and new perspectives to emerge in your mind. Once you have opened your mind to novel ideas, you can reintroduce your critical modes of thought to evaluate what you have discovered and to decide on an appropriate course of action (using the problem-solving and decision-making methods described above).

Since creativity involves taking risks with your own thought processes, you need to be able to do this while tolerating the discomfort that it may very well involve. The subject of creativity is so large as to warrant a text to itself and, indeed, several useful books have been written on the subject. I recommend that the interested reader should consult Roger von Oech's interesting book *A Whack on the Side of the Head* (Warner Books, 1998).

Step 8

Develop and pursue vitally absorbing interests

Like all human beings, you are likely to be at your happiest when you are pursuing a vitally absorbing, personally meaningful interest. In contrast, you easily get bored and discouraged with routine, everyday, mundane activity which is neither vitally absorbing nor personally meaningful. Thus, if you are to strive to be mentally healthy, you need to identify a number of interests, projects and activities which are both personally meaningful to you and vitally absorbing, so that you can become not only happy but mentally healthy.

In Step 5, I made the point that as a unique, complex individual, you are going to have unique and complex preferences. The same point holds true when you consider your vitally absorbing interests. Discover what is personally meaningful to you and, as long as it does not significantly interfere with the interests of your significant others and is unlikely to do other people harm, actively pursue those interests no matter how idiosyncratic they are and no matter how absurd they may appear to other people.

Human beings are such that they are frequently intolerant of other people's interests that they consider to be different from their own. Thus, a man who is vitally absorbed in opera will find it 'ridiculous' that another man can be vitally absorbed in train spotting. No doubt the train spotter will have similar views about the opera buff. Thus, if you are to throw yourself into your vitally absorbing interest, you may need to develop a reasonably thick skin when it comes to the views of others, otherwise you might experience a lot of shame if other people were to discover your unique and idiosyncratic interests. This may discourage you from actively pursuing your interests, or you may do so with an underlying sense of shame.

Overcoming shame

In this context, shame is an emotion that stems, like other emotions, from a philosophy towards yourself with respect to how you are viewed by others. Let's take the example of the train spotter. If other people pour scorn on train spotting, what would he (in this case) have to tell himself in order to feel ashamed? He would need to tell himself:

1 'Other people think my train spotting is strange.' This inference may well be true. Not everybody will but some definitely will.
2 'Because other people find my interest strange, they think that I am a strange person.' This is probably an arrant overgeneralization and will frequently be untrue. There are, no doubt, some people who, because they find your interest strange, will foolishly conclude that you are a completely strange person, but most people will not do this. So, if the train spotter finds himself thinking in this way, he needs to identify the distortion and correct it using the methods described in the previous step.
3 'If other people find me strange and shameful, they're right, I am.' This is the essence of shame, because even if the train spotter made Stages 1 and 2 above, he would not feel ashamed if he accepted himself at Stage 3. For this reason I would advise the train spotter to assume temporarily that his inferences in Stages 1 and 2 are true so that he can identify and challenge his underlying shame-creating philosophy.

How should our train spotter overcome his shame? First, he needs to ask himself questions like: 'How does it follow that if other people think I'm strange and shameful, this proves that I really am strange?' He can then answer the question thus: 'Even if other people do make such foolish overgeneralizations, I can never be shameful because I am far too complex an individual to merit such a label. If I really was a shameful individual, everything about me would be shameful and this is completely ridiculous. Thus, I am a fallible human being who has interests that some people find strange; this is unfortunate and I had better accept this grim reality and pursue my vitally absorbing interests nonetheless.'

Using this question-and-answer method, you can help yourself considerably by minimizing the shame in your life as you actively pursue your own interests.

The importance of activity

As I mentioned at the beginning of this step, human beings seem to be happier being actively involved in some vitally absorbing interest than being passively involved. Thus, it is important that you throw yourself into the interests that you find personally meaningful and vitally absorbing. You need to counter any tendency that you may have to be passive in the pursuit of your real interests.

As noted in Step 4, becoming actively involved in something meaningful, and sustaining your activity in your interest, requires that you develop greater discomfort tolerance. Thus, I suggest that you review the points I made in that step if you consider that discomfort intolerance is a problem for you in this area. However, discomfort intolerance is likely to be less of a problem in these circumstances, primarily because your vitally absorbing interest is just that – vital and absorbing. Thus, you often find sufficient interest in the activity to motivate yourself to be active. However, there is no doubt that some aspects of actively pursuing your vitally absorbing interest are likely to be tedious and a hassle, and it is here that your discomfort intolerance beliefs may hold you back. As such, you need to identify, challenge and change the following two discomfort intolerance beliefs.

'It's too much hassle to do this today, I'll put it off until tomorrow' Here you need to show yourself that you are jumping from rating the activity as a hassle, which it may well be, to it being *too* much of a hassle, which it most certainly isn't. This stems from an underlying demand that life conditions must not be as hard as they are. You need to challenge this rigid belief not only in your mind but through action that is inconsistent with it. Thus, you could literally show yourself, through action, that the tedious activity involved in pursuing your interest is a hassle but that it is worth doing. Also, don't forget that procrastination is, in such circumstances, a

delusion, because it is unlikely that the activity is going to become less of a hassle tomorrow.

'I'll wait until I feel like doing it' If you wait until you feel like doing a tedious aspect of your vitally absorbing interest, you may wait for a very long time indeed. Note that throwing yourself into the aspect that you do not feel like doing can lead you to minimize its tedious aspects, while if you wait until you feel like doing it, you often build up the tediousness of the task in your mind. In addition, if you throw yourself into something that you do not feel like doing at a particular time, you may well find that this feeling soon passes and that you become involved in the activity sooner than you predicted you would.

Even though discomfort intolerance issues are less likely to be involved in your pursuit of your vitally absorbing interests than in other areas of your life, don't conclude that therefore they will definitely not occur. So look out for ways in which you stop yourself from becoming as actively involved in your real interests as you can and deal effectively with these obstacles.

Be devoted without being devout

One of the dangers of pursuing a vitally absorbing interest is that you become devout or dogmatic about it. You may literally become addicted to the interest at the expense of your other interests, your job and your personal relationships, all of which suffer as you rigidly follow your own nose. When this happens you are like a horse with blinkers on. The only thing you can see or think about is your vitally absorbing interest. A devout approach to pursuing interests seems to be based on a number of irrational beliefs. You may believe that because your interest is particularly fascinating, you must pursue it at every available opportunity. Correspondingly, you may believe that it would be awful to be deprived of your vitally absorbing activity and that you cannot stand being away from it for very long. You may also falsely consider yourself to be a more worthwhile person when you are involved in the activity, particularly if you are doing well at it. So if being devout rather than being devoted to your special interest is a problem for you –

and you will find this out because other people will frequently bring it to your attention – look for your underlying irrational beliefs. In particular, look for your rigid beliefs, awfulizing beliefs, discomfort intolerance beliefs and, paradoxically, positively evaluating yourself when you are involved in the activity and negatively evaluating yourself when you are not. Identify these beliefs as specifically as you can and challenge them in ways that I have already described in this book and will consider in greater depth in Step 10.

Becoming devoutly involved in a vitally absorbing interest, as opposed to being devoted to it, can also be a sign that you have a problem in your life which you are attempting to cover up by inflexibly involving yourself in your chosen activity. Many years ago, a female friend told me a sad story about what happened to her when she and her husband had a baby. Before the baby arrived, they were a loving couple; the husband had a special interest in train spotting but it did not interfere with his marriage. Thus, he was devoted to it, but not devoutly so. However, as soon as the baby was born, his interest in trains increased markedly. At every possible moment he would head for shunting yards in pursuit of numbers of trains that he had not yet collected. It transpired that this man was extraordinarily jealous of the baby's arrival and felt that he was displaced from his wife's affection. Rather than confronting this problem and working it through with her, he pushed it to one side and tried to solve the problem through his now devout involvement in train spotting. If you suspect that your involvement in your vitally absorbing interest is getting out of hand, and that you are becoming dogmatic about it, ask yourself whether you are using it to cover up problems in your life. If this is so, read my book *Transforming Eight Deadly Emotions into Healthy Ones* (Sheldon Press, 2012), which may give you some idea about how to solve your emotional problems. If further help is required, please do not hesitate to seek counselling. Either consult your GP or, for a list of counsellors and psychotherapists in your area, write to the British Association for Counselling and Psychotherapy, BACP House, 15 St John's Business Park, Lutterworth, Leicestershire LE17 4HB (<www.bacp.co.uk>).

Experiment

What if you do not have a vitally absorbing interest at the moment, or if an interest is becoming less vital for you? The best answer that I know to this problem can be summed up in one word – experiment. Adopting an experimental attitude towards new interests that may become vitally absorbing for you of course involves risks. It may well be that you will be spending time on interests and activities that, in the long run, do not hold your interest. This is a risk that you need to accept if you are to benefit in the long term from experimenting. If you will only devote time to such experimentation if things work out in the end, you will not allow yourself to experiment with new interests and activities. You don't have a crystal ball. How can you tell whether the expenditure of time and effort and energy is going to be worth it in the long run? The short answer is, you don't. However, you may wish to save *some* time by finding out as much information as you can about a proposed activity and by imagining yourself becoming involved in it. Using your mind's eye in this way can sometimes lead you to conclude accurately that an activity is not for you. However, numerous people have been pleasantly surprised by finding that they have really enjoyed an activity that they thought they would not enjoy. So, even though you may think that you will not gain pleasure out of an activity, it may still be worth your while experimenting with it.

How long should you give a new activity before you conclude that it's not for you? In some circumstances it will be clear right from the start. However, with other activities you may need to give them a bit more time. Some activities are an acquired taste and it takes some time before you acquire it. Why not (flexibly) apply what I call the baseball rule? In baseball, a batter is struck out if three correct pitches are delivered against him. Thus, if you find that after three *serious* attempts at an activity you are not getting some enjoyment out of it, then the activity is probably not for you. Be mindful, however, that I have emphasized making three *serious* attempts. If you make half-hearted attempts at anything, then it is unlikely that you will get the information you need to determine whether or not an activity has the potential to become a vitally absorbing one for you.

Step 9

Improve your relationships with others

Many research studies show quite clearly the important effects that having good relationships with others have on one's mental health. Indeed, it would be difficult to imagine someone being mentally healthy who also had poor or superficial relationships with others, or in fact conducted his or her life away from other people. I suppose there are a small number of hermits who may be mentally healthy, but they are very much the exception. In consequence, if you wish to be mentally healthy, it is important that you improve your relationships with other human beings.

Unconditionally accepting other people

A central plank on which to base your improved relationships with others is one that involves you adopting an unconditional acceptance belief with respect to other people. This means being flexible in your preferences about others and refraining from being rigid about the way these others should be. It means recognizing that other people may well frustrate your desires, but that this is unfortunate rather than awful. It involves building up your level of discomfort tolerance when you come into conflict with others as a prelude to working these conflicts through. It involves you developing unconditional acceptance of others, which recognizes that they too are fallible human beings who are a complex mixture of good, bad and neutral.

If you are able to apply such an accepting philosophy to others, you will then be able to tolerate differences between yourself and other people. In my many years' work counselling couples, this ability to tolerate differences between oneself and one's partner is, for me, a powerful predictor of a good marriage. When you fail to accept that your partner may have different views on important issues or may have different interests and tastes, it is very easy to then make the demand that he or she must not be the way he or she is. This attitude is the breeding ground for much interpersonal conflict between partners.

Therefore, it is important to cultivate tolerance for the differences that there will inevitably be between yourself and others. If you are able to celebrate your own uniqueness as discussed in Step 5, you will be in a better position to celebrate the uniqueness of your partner, for example. Being able to do so is an important part of developing respect for your partner and, if you can generalize this respectful attitude towards others, this will stand you in very good stead to cultivate good relationships with them.

Develop a healthy trusting attitude towards others

Trust is a very difficult issue for so many people today. I define trust as a sense of confidence that somebody will not take significant advantage of you. However, given that other people are also fallible human beings, it is not beyond the realms of possibility that they will do so, given the fact that they have their own problems and human failings.

In my experience, the problems that people have in trusting other people fall into two main categories. First of all, there are those who have a naive faith in other people. If you are such a person, you believe implicitly that other people with whom you come into contact will not harm or take advantage of you. You thus end up frequently being taken advantage of because you fail to discriminate between those who are trustworthy and those who are not. If you place your trust naively in others, you believe that they are caring individuals who will all go out of their way to be kind and helpful to you. It is important for you to give up your naivety and learn to discriminate, on the basis of experience, between those people who can be trusted (although not in an absolute sense) and those who cannot be so trusted.

The second and, in my experience, by far the most common group have difficulty trusting other people because they are deeply suspicious of them. If you are such a person you will commonly say that you find it difficult getting close to people because you do not want to end up being treated badly (or, more colloquially, being hurt). As such you hold two related beliefs. First, you believe that you must have a guarantee that you won't be hurt before you start trusting somebody and, second, you believe it would be absolutely terrible to be hurt. Rather than face this possibility, you decide that it is far better to develop only superficial relationships with other people. Since your superficial relationships with others are basically unsatisfying, although for you less frightening, than more intimate relationships, you are caught in a trap between being comfortable and unsatisfied, on the one hand, and being frightened by the prospect of intimacy, on the other.

In order to develop a healthy sense of trust in others, you need to dispute the idea that you must have a guarantee that you will not be hurt. As with other guarantees, guaranteed immunity from being let down or hurt is simply not obtainable. Even if another person promises explicitly that she will never hurt you, this does not constitute a guarantee, since the other person is basically a human being with problems, weaknesses and failings, and these may well lead her to act in a way which may be at times hurtful to you.

You also need to challenge the belief that you must not be let down or betrayed and it would be terrible if you were. Let me be quite clear on this point. Being let down and betrayed is a very unpleasant experience which nobody would actively seek out. Far from it. However, once you are dealing with other human beings, it is important to recognize that this may happen at times. Surrendering your awfulizing belief about being let down or hurt, and giving up your demand that this absolutely must not happen, is the key to developing a more sensible, trusting relationship with other people.

If you have a healthy, trusting attitude towards other people, you will then be far better placed to evaluate how badly you have been let down or betrayed. For example, if you believe that it is important for you to be in a monogamous relationship with a loved one and this loved one is unfaithful to you, you may conclude that your relationship with this person is at an end. However, you might decide to give this person a second chance, only ending the relationship if you are betrayed again.

If you are a naive, trusting individual, you may be far too toler-ant of your loved one's peccadillos, with the result that you may be continually betrayed, whereas if you are basically suspicious in the area of trust, you may not only decide to end the relationship, but you may also decide never to enter another relationship again.

If you have a healthy, trusting attitude towards people, you will take due care and concern to discriminate between people whom you can trust and those people whom it may be sensible to stay away from. The important points here are that you are flexible in your decisions and that you let your experiences guide these deci-sions rather than your too-trusting or unduly suspicious attitudes.

Communicate caringly

Caring communication towards others involves you communicat-ing both your positive and your negative feelings. There is an abun-dance of texts on assertion. While these books give some attention to the communication of your positive feelings, they mainly deal with how you can best communicate your negative feelings and stand up for your rights. However, if you are to develop healthy relationships with other people, then you need to place more emphasis on the communication of your positive feelings towards them than your negative feelings.

Communicate your positive feelings

If you want to develop good relationships with other people, it is important that you tell them what you like both about them and about what they have done. Do this from the position of accept-ing them as fallible human beings who are composed of positive, negative and neutral attributes. Do not imply that you like them more if they do well and therefore less if they do poorly. Say such things as: 'I appreciate what you did for me'; 'I like the way you said that'; 'I think you're doing a really good job'; 'I really like the fact that you are going out of your way to help other people.'

As Dale Carnegie noted in his best-selling book *How to Win Friends and Influence People*, it is crucial that your positive com-munications to other people are genuine. If you put on an act, sooner or later people will see through this and it will rebound on you. Thus, only communicate your positive feelings if they are genuinely felt. Even if you are the type of person who is over-critical, it is possible to train yourself to look for aspects of other people's behaviour that you like or appreciate. Once you have found these, do not hesitate to communicate your appreciation. Being on the receiving end of such positive communications, though initially embarrassing, will be appreciated and certainly not forgotten. Communicating positively to other people will help you greatly in encouraging them to feel positively towards you.

How to communicate your negative feelings

In my book *The Incredible Sulk* (Sheldon Press, 1992), I outlined eight steps to healthy self-assertion when you need to communicate your negative feelings to other people.

1 Get the person's attention It is no good trying to assert yourself with another person if he (in this case) is preoccupied. Therefore, before you proceed to communicate your negative feelings, ensure that he is listening to you with as much attention as he can muster.

2 Describe objectively the other person's behaviour that you do not like When you bring to the attention of another person that you do not like some aspect of his behaviour, then it is very important that you do so in as objective a way as possible. Do not make inferences and do not cast aspersions on the other person's character. Say, 'I don't like the fact that you said that about me', rather than 'I don't like the fact that you criticized me.' The latter is an inference whereas the former is an objective description.

3 Communicate your healthy negative feelings In this book I have distinguished between healthy negative feelings and unhealthy negative feelings. At this point in the communication process, it is crucial for you to communicate your healthy negative feelings and not your unhealthy negative feelings. If you communicate your unhealthy negative feelings, you will encourage the other person to become over-defensive and this will interfere with your constructive relationship with him. Thus, communicate your sorrow or your healthy anger rather than your feelings of hurt or unhealthy anger. When you communicate your feelings of hurt and unhealthy anger, you increase the chances that the other person will respond offensively or defensively, whereas if you communicate your feelings of sorrow and healthy anger, the other person will be more inclined to listen to you.

4 Check your inferences and invite a response It is difficult for human beings to avoid making inferences about another person's behaviour. However, you need to realize that your inferences are hunches about reality rather than facts. Therefore, when you communicate your inference to another person, put it as a hunch rather than as a fact and check with the other person whether or not he thinks you have a point. Then, invite him to make a response.

5 Listen to the other person's response and give feedback Once you have invited the other person to make a response, show him respect by listening to him without interruption. If you interrupt him while he is communicating to you, even though you do not like what he is saying, this is more likely to make him defensive and to interfere with your constructive relationship with him. However, if you listen to the other person without interruption, he has a sense that he has been heard and listened to. You are then in a better position to give any constructive feedback on what he has said.

6 State your flexible preferences clearly and explicitly After you have listened to the other person and given initial feedback, it is important that you communicate clearly what you want from him (e.g. a different response from the one that he has previously given you). Remind yourself, and also the other person, if appropriate, that you do not *have to* get what you want, even though you are perfectly entitled to want it. Therefore, make sure that you have communicated clearly so that the other person has understood what it is that you are looking for. If you assume, for example, that the person must know what you are looking for, then you are engaging in an unhelpful form of mind-reading and this will over-complicate your relationship with the other person.

7 Request agreement from the other person After you have communicated your flexible preference, ask for feedback from the other person and, more specifically, seek agreement from him that he is prepared to do what you have requested. If he is not prepared to make such an agreement, then you may need to engage him in further assertive communication.

8 Communicate any relevant information concerning future episodes
This final step in the self-assertive sequence involves you communicating any relevant information that you want the other person to have concerning future similar episodes. Thus, you might say, 'The next time this happens, I'll be sure to mention my feelings to you at that time', or 'The next time this happens, how would you like me to bring this to your attention?' This latter communication is specifically relevant when the other person claims that he does not realize that he is acting in a negative manner.

This process of assertive communication is a central feature of developing a healthy negotiating style with another person so that you can minimize conflict with him or her. It will also be more likely to lead to healthy compromise and conciliation. Making compromises is important if you are to continue a relationship with that other person; its purpose is to ensure that you both get something out of continued interaction with one another. If this is not done, then your continued relationship will be marked by an undercurrent of unexpressed resentment. This is conducive neither to your mental health nor to that of the other person.

Honour your commitments to others

An important part of demonstrating that you are trustworthy in relationships is for you to keep your promises. This is an important aspect of interpersonal relationships which, in my opinion, is sadly neglected in psychology texts on the subject. Honouring your commitments to others means that it is important for you to follow through in doing what you say you are prepared to do, even though more attractive options may crop up in the interim. It is here that you need to practise your developing discomfort tolerance.

For example, if John agreed to take Mary to a play in a week's time, how should John handle the situation when a more attractive social invitation comes his way? My view is that John needs to tell himself something like, 'I have promised to take Mary to the

play and I am going to do so, even though it might be more enjoyable for me to attend this other social engagement. If I let Mary
down, then this may prejudice our future relationship with one
another and I do not want this to happen. Therefore, I am going
to put up with the frustration of missing out on this new social
engagement and to be pleased that I am demonstrating my commitment to my relationship with Mary.'

If you want to elicit trust from other people, one of the best ways
of doing this is to show them that you are prepared to honour your
commitments to them, that you are reliable and that you will not
allow passing whims to prevent you from keeping your promises.
This means that when you tell someone that you will telephone
her at a given time, you undertake to do so, even though this may
mean breaking off an enjoyable activity. Sustaining interpersonal
relationships involves putting up with discomfort and frustration;
it also involves forgoing pleasures that may be immediately very
gratifying. However, if you want to sustain good relationships with
other people, this is what you need to do.

Develop social interests

In Step 5, I argued that it was important for you to develop an
attitude of self-care (sometimes called enlightened self-interest). I
contrasted this attitude with one of selfishness; the former dem-
onstrates that you are basically interested in yourself but also, and
fundamentally so, in the well-being of other people, particularly
those who are significant to you. Selfishness, however, is based on
an attitude that you must always come first; other people's desires
are unimportant and can be easily neglected. Therefore, if you wish
to improve your relationships with other people, it is important to
develop a real interest in their well-being as well as in your own.
This involves being sensitive to other people's wishes and trying
to meet them, unless doing so conflicts with your own important
desires. Sometimes this may involve putting other people's desires
above your own when their wishes are more important to them
than yours are to you.

Nurturing other people involves not only communicating to
them verbally that you care for them and are interested in them,

but also demonstrating this through your actions. Here, one caring action will speak louder than a thousand caring words. Also, if you nurture others you will find that they are more likely to nurture you.

From a wider perspective, demonstrating social interest involves you helping your immediate circle of significant others, a wider circle of people who live in your community and also others who need help in far-flung corners of the world. The more you help other people who are in need, the more you will feel centrally involved in both the world's affairs in general and your immediate circle of significant others in particular.

Develop healthy interdependencies

In my experience, good interpersonal relationships are formed when people become interdependent. This means that they are willing to help one another when they are in need and that this is a two-way process. There are three other positions which are relevant here, which, in my experience, interfere with good interpersonal relationships.

Dependency

When you are dependent on another person, you become anxious if that person is not around to help you and care for you, or worry that your relationship with him or her may be interrupted (which you, in your dependent state, will see as abandonment). Dependency is based on a rigid belief that you need other people on whom to rely and on the idea that you have poor coping skills to survive happily on your own. Relationships which are characterized by dependency tend to be unsatisfactory for both partners. The dependent person comes to hate himself for his own weakness, and the non-dependent person comes to resent the almost claustrophobic relationship that develops between the two of them. So, if you recognize that you tend to be a dependent person, accept yourself unconditionally for your dependency, identify the irrational beliefs that underpin your dependency, and work towards a more healthy, independent position which will then enable you to participate in healthy interdependent relationships.

Compulsive helping

Frequently, people who are dependent tend to develop relationships with those who gain strength from nurturing dependent people. While the dependent person needs to be needed, the compulsive helper, as I call such a person, needs to help others and therefore needs to be needed by others. Frequently, compulsive helpers gain strength from tending to other seemingly helpless individuals. However, if you scratch the surface of compulsive helpers, you frequently find that they are covering up their own weaknesses by adopting a seemingly strong position of helping the other person. So, if you are somebody who can recognize compulsive helping tendencies in yourself, look for and acknowledge your intolerance of your own weaknesses. Accept yourself unconditionally with your weaknesses, deal with them and then develop more equal, interdependent relationships, rather than a relationship where you are in the one-up position of being a compulsive helper, aiding others who are in the one-down position of dependency.

Compulsive self-reliance

The third position that I wish to discuss here has been called compulsive self-reliance by the well-known pioneer of attachment theory John Bowlby. If you are compulsively self-reliant, you gain self-worth from being able to solve all your own problems without involving another person. While the compulsive helper gains strength from helping another person, the compulsively self-reliant person gains strength in being able to help himself or herself and from not seeking help from another person. Compulsively self-reliant people tend to shun intimate relationships or, if they involve themselves in these relationships, are soon criticized for not sharing their vulnerabil-ities with their partners. People who are compulsively self-reliant are underlyingly shameful about their weaknesses and believe that they can overcome their shame by being even more strong. However, their interpersonal relationships tend to suffer, either because they become shallow or because they withdraw into themselves, a position from which they neither nurture their partner nor seek nurturance from their partner.

If you recognize that you are compulsively self-reliant, it is important for you to challenge the belief which states that you are a shameful, weak person if you have vulnerabilities. Then, from this developing new belief of unconditional self-acceptance, take risks and share your vulnerabilities with your partner and develop an increasingly interdependent relationship, which is the epitome of mental health for both partners who are lucky enough to experience such a relationship.

Step 10

Develop a realistic outlook on personal change

An important aspect of developing mental health is adopting a realistic outlook on personal change. In this final step, I will outline 11 stages that you need to go through if you wish to embark on a realistic self-change programme.

Stage 1: Admit that you have a problem and accept yourself for it It is difficult to change a problem if you are unprepared to admit to it. One of the blocks to admitting a problem includes being ashamed about having the problem. Here you believe, 'If I admit I have this problem, this will prove what a worthless, inadequate, weak, incapable person I am.' Believing this, it is easier to deny that you have a problem and to blame other people for your problem than to admit that you have a problem. So, an important aspect of admitting a problem involves accepting yourself for having it. As I showed you in Step 5 of this book, an important feature of being mentally healthy is to develop unconditional self-acceptance. You do not see yourself as being more worthy if you did not have it or less worthy because you do have it. Admitting that you have a problem enables you to accept responsibility for it, and this will enable you to go to the next stage in your self-change programme.

Stage 2: Be specific It is very difficult to overcome problems which are quite vague in nature. So be as specific as you can, not only when you outline what your problem is but when you take an example to analyse.

Stage 3: Identify your disturbed emotion The more you can specify what your disturbed emotion is, the more likely it is that you will understand what you are disturbed about. Try to avoid writing down such statements as 'I feel upset' or 'I feel distressed'. Also, realize that not all negative emotions are unhealthy. For example, you may be experiencing healthy sadness in response to a loss, healthy concern in response to a threat, healthy anger in response to some frustration; in general, because of their healthy nature, these are not emotional problems. However, if you regard them as being problems, you probably believe that you should not feel negative at all in such circumstances. You may believe, for example, that faced with a threat you should be calm, or faced with a loss you should be stoical, or faced with an insult you should turn the other cheek. So, ensure that you write down feelings like anxiety, depression, guilt, shame, unhealthy anger, hurt or self-pity, unhealthy jealousy and unhealthy envy, which are all clearly both negative and self-defeating in nature.

Stage 4: Identify the aspect of the situation that you are most disturbed about When you are feeling a negative unhealthy emotion (as discussed above), it is important to focus on what you are most disturbed about. When you are in a particular situation, you are faced with several different aspects about which you could be disturbed. So the more you can pinpoint the aspect of the situation that you are most anxious about, for example, the more you are going to be able to help yourself in a realistic manner.

Let's suppose that you are anxious about speaking in public. It could be that you are anxious in case you stammer. It could be that you are anxious about the possibility of drying up. You may be anxious that your audience will take pity on you, or you may be anxious that the audience may be overcritical of you. The more you can focus on what you are most disturbed about, the better. So, ask yourself, 'What was it about this situation that I was most anxious about?' This is the element towards which you need to develop a new rational belief.

Sometimes it will be obvious that the aspect of the situation that you are most disturbed about is clearly distorted. For example, you may decide that you are scared that the members of the audience are all going to get up and walk out. Now this is very unlikely, but since it is what you are scared about, it is important at this point to assume temporarily that it will happen. This will enable you to identify your unhelpful, irrational beliefs, which constitutes Stage 5.

Stage 5: Identify your irrational beliefs As noted in Steps 2 to 5 of this book, there are four irrational beliefs that underpin much human emotional disturbance.

- A rigid belief: here, you believe that you, other people and the world must be or not be a certain way.
- An awfulizing belief: here, you believe that it would be awful, terrible and the end of the world if the conditions that you insist must exist do not occur.
- A discomfort intolerance belief: here, you believe that if the situation that you demand must not occur actually occurred, then you would not be able to tolerate it. This means that you would either die on the spot or never experience happiness again.
- A depreciation belief with respect to self, others and the world: here, you believe that you are less worthy under certain conditions – that if another person blocks you, for example, that person is damnable and that the world is rotten for allowing bad things to happen to you or others.

Look for the presence of one or more of these beliefs and appreciate that it is these beliefs that are primarily responsible for your disturbed feelings.

Stage 6: Develop rational alternatives to your irrational beliefs Before you question your irrational beliefs, it is important that you construct rational alternatives to these beliefs. This is important for the following reasons:

- Constructing a set of rational alternative beliefs gives you something constructive to believe in.
- If you don't have something to aim for with respect to your beliefs you will go back to your irrational beliefs, since humans do not function well in a belief vacuum.

- Rational beliefs underpin a constructive set of responses to adversities and point to how you can best achieve these constructive goals.

Thus, construct the following rational beliefs as appropriate:

- A flexible belief: here, you believe that while you may want yourself, other people and the world to be a certain way, it does not follow that you, others and the world have to be that way.
- A non-awfulizing belief: here, you believe that while it would be bad if the conditions that you desire did not exist, it is not the end of the world if they don't.
- A discomfort tolerance belief: here, you believe that if the situation that you desire did not occur, then while it would be a struggle you would be able to tolerate it and it would be in your interests to do so.
- An unconditional acceptance belief with respect to self, others and the world: here, you believe that you are the same fallible human being under changing conditions – that if another person blocks you, for example, that person is fallible and not damnable and the world is not rotten for allowing bad things to happen to you or others. Rather, it is a complex mixture of the good, the bad and the neutral.

Stage 7: Question your irrational and rational beliefs There are three main ways of questioning irrational and rational beliefs. The first way is to ask questions concerning how consistent the belief is with reality. The second way is to ask questions concerning the logic of the belief. The third way is to ask questions of the consequences of holding the belief.

I suggest that you question your rational and irrational beliefs together and question each of the four pairs one at a time.

In Tables 10.1, 10.2, 10.3 and 10.4 (on the following pages), I give suggestions concerning reasons why the four irrational beliefs are false, illogical and largely unhealthy and why the four alternative rational beliefs are true, logical and largely healthy.

Table 10.1 Reasons why rigid beliefs are false, illogical and have largely unhealthy consequences and flexible beliefs are true, logical and have largely healthy consequences

Rigid belief	Flexible belief

A rigid belief is false

For such a demand to be true the demanded conditions would already have to exist when they do not, or as soon as you make a demand then these demanded conditions would have to come into existence. Both positions are clearly false or inconsistent with reality.

A flexible belief is true

A flexible belief is true because its two component parts are true. You can prove that you have a particular desire and can provide reasons why you want what you want. You can also prove that you do not have to get what you desire.

A rigid belief is illogical

A rigid belief is based on the same desire as a flexible belief but is transformed as follows:

'I prefer that x happens (or does not happen) . . . and therefore this absolutely must (or must not) happen.'

The first – 'I prefer that x happens (or does not happen) . . .' – is not rigid, but the second – '. . . and therefore this must (or must not) happen' – is rigid. As such, a rigid belief is illogical since one cannot logically derive something rigid from something that is not rigid.

A flexible belief is logical

A flexible belief is logical since both parts are not rigid and thus the second component logically follows from the first. Thus, consider the following flexible belief:

'I prefer that x happens (or does not happen) . . . but this does not mean that it must (or must not) happen.'

The first component – 'I prefer that x happens (or does not happen) . . .' – is not rigid, and the second – '. . . but this does not mean that it must (or must not) happen' – is also non-rigid. Thus, a flexible belief is logical because it is comprised of two non-rigid parts connected together logically.

A rigid belief has largely unhealthy consequences

A rigid belief has largely unhealthy consequences because it tends to lead to unhealthy negative emotions, unconstructive behaviour and highly distorted and biased subsequent thinking when you are facing an adversity.

A flexible belief has largely healthy consequences

A flexible belief has largely healthy consequences because it tends to lead to healthy negative emotions, constructive behaviour and realistic and balanced subsequent thinking when you are facing an adversity.

Table 10.2 Reasons why awfulizing beliefs are false, illogical and have largely unhealthy consequences and non-awfulizing beliefs are true, logical and have largely healthy consequences

Awfulizing belief	*Non-awfulizing belief*
An awfulizing belief is false When you hold an awfulizing belief about your adversity, this belief is based on the following ideas: 1 Nothing could be worse. 2 The event in question is worse than 100 per cent bad. 3 No good could possibly come from this bad event. All three ideas are patently false and thus your awfulizing belief is false.	**A non-awfulizing belief is true** When you hold a non-awfulizing belief about your adversity, this belief is based on the following ideas: 1 Things could always be worse. 2 The event in question is less than 100 per cent bad. 3 Good could come from this bad event. All three ideas are clearly true and thus your non-awfulizing belief is true.
An awfulizing belief is illogical An awfulizing belief is based on the same evaluation of badness as a non-awfulizing belief but is transformed as follows: *'It is bad if x happens (or does not happen) . . . .and therefore it is awful if it does happen (or does not happen).'* The first component – 'It is bad if x happens (or does not happen) . . .' – is non-extreme, but the second – '. . . and therefore it is awful if it does (or does not) happen' – is extreme. As such, an awfulizing belief is illogical since one cannot logically derive something extreme from something that is non-extreme.	**A non-awfulizing belief is logical** A non-awfulizing belief is logical since both parts are non-extreme, and thus the second component logically follows from the first. Thus, consider the following non-awfulizing belief: *'It is bad if x happens (or does not happen) . . . but it is not awful if x happens (or does not happen).'* The first component – 'It is bad if x happens (or does not happen) . . .' – is non-extreme, and the second – '. . . but it is not awful if it does (or does not happen)' – is also non-extreme. Thus, a non-awfulizing belief is logical because it is comprised of two non-extreme parts connected together logically.
An awfulizing belief has largely unhealthy consequences An awfulizing belief has largely unhealthy consequences because it tends to lead to unhealthy negative emotions, unconstructive behaviour and highly distorted and biased subsequent thinking when you are facing an adversity.	**A non-awfulizing belief has largely healthy consequences** A non-awfulizing belief has largely healthy consequences because it tends to lead to healthy negative emotions, constructive behaviour and realistic and balanced subsequent thinking when you are facing an adversity.

Table 10.3 Reasons why discomfort intolerance beliefs are false, illogical and have largely unhealthy consequences and discomfort tolerance beliefs are true, logical and have largely healthy consequences

Discomfort intolerance belief	Discomfort tolerance belief
A discomfort intolerance belief is false When you hold a discomfort intolerance belief about your adversity, this belief is based on the following ideas, which are all false: 1 I will die or disintegrate if the discomfort continues to exist. 2 I will lose the capacity to experience happiness if the discomfort continues to exist. 3 Even if I could tolerate it, the discomfort is not worth tolerating. All three ideas are patently false and thus your discomfort intolerance belief is false.	**A discomfort tolerance belief is true** When you hold a discomfort tolerance belief about your adversity, this belief is based on the following ideas, which are all true: 1 I will struggle if the discomfort continues to exist, but I will neither die nor disintegrate. 2 I will not lose the capacity to experience happiness if the discomfort continues to exist, although this capacity will be temporarily diminished. 3 The discomfort is worth tolerating. All three ideas are patently true and thus your discomfort tolerance belief is true.
A discomfort intolerance belief is illogical A discomfort intolerance belief is based on the same sense of struggle as a discomfort tolerance belief, but is transformed as follows: *'It would be difficult for me to tolerate it if x happened (or did not happen) and therefore it would be intolerable.'* The first component – 'It would be difficult for me to tolerate it if x happened (or did not happen) . . .' – is non-extreme, but the second –'. . . and therefore it would be intolerable' – is extreme. As such, a discomfort intolerance belief is illogical since one cannot logically derive something extreme from something that is non-extreme.	**A discomfort tolerance belief is logical** A discomfort tolerance belief is logical, since both parts are non-extreme and thus the second component logically follows from the first. Thus, consider the following discomfort tolerance belief: *'It would be difficult for me to tolerate it if x happened (or did not happen) but it would not be intolerable (and it would be worth tolerating).'* The first component – 'It would be difficult for me to tolerate it if x happened (or did not happen) . . .' – is non-extreme and the second – '. . . but it would not be intolerable (and it would be worth tolerating)' – is also non-extreme. Thus, a discomfort tolerance belief is logical because it is comprised of two non-extreme parts connected together logically.

A discomfort intolerance belief has largely unhealthy consequences	A discomfort tolerance belief has largely healthy consequences
A discomfort intolerance belief has largely unhealthy consequences because it tends to lead to unhealthy negative emotions, unconstructive behaviour and highly distorted and biased subsequent thinking when you are facing an adversity.	A discomfort tolerance belief has largely healthy consequences because it tends to lead to healthy negative emotions, constructive behaviour and realistic and balanced subsequent thinking when you are facing an adversity.

Stage 8: Practise strengthening your rational beliefs Your four main rational beliefs, if you recall, are:

- a flexible belief with respect to your desires;
- a non-awfulizing belief;
- a discomfort tolerance belief;
- an unconditional acceptance belief with respect to self, others and the world.

The important point to recognize here is that you will not develop conviction in these rational beliefs until you practise acting on them regularly and forcefully. Acting on your new rational beliefs once or twice a week in an unconvincing, half-hearted manner isn't going to strengthen them, but frequent practice at acting on the rational beliefs in a strong, fully committed manner will. So, make a commitment to do so and watch out for the five major traps that may stop you from acting on your new rational beliefs in a fully committed and regular manner.

- *'I cannot take constructive action until I am comfortable.'* If you wait until you are comfortable, you will wait for a very long time before taking such constructive action. So, act on your new rational beliefs even though it is uncomfortable to do so. You will become more comfortable later, after much practice.
- *'I cannot take constructive action because I do not have a sense of control.'* Once again, it is important to act even though you may feel out of control, because the more you act on your new rational beliefs, the more you will strengthen your sense of control.

Table 10.4 Reasons why depreciation beliefs are false, illogical and have largely unhealthy consequences and acceptance beliefs are true, logical and have largely healthy consequences

Depreciation belief	Acceptance belief
A depreciation belief is false When you hold a depreciation belief in the face of your adversity, this belief is based on the following ideas, which are all false: 1 A person (self or other) or life can legitimately be given a single global rating that defines his or her or its essence and the worth of a person or of life is dependent upon conditions that change (e.g. 'my worth goes up when I do well and goes down when I don't do well'). 2 A person or life can be rated on the basis of one of his or her or its aspects. Both of these ideas are patently false and thus your depreciation belief is false.	**An acceptance belief is true** When you hold an acceptance belief in the face of your adversity, this belief is based on the following ideas, which are all true: 1 A person (self or other) or life cannot legitimately be given a single global rating that defines the person's or life's essence, and the worth of that person or of life, as far as such worth exists, is not dependent upon conditions that change (e.g. 'my worth stays the same whether or not I do well'). 2 Discrete aspects of a person and life can be legitimately rated, but a person or life cannot be legitimately rated on the basis of these discrete aspects. Both of these ideas are patently true and thus your acceptance belief is true.
A depreciation belief is illogical A depreciation belief is based on the idea that the whole of a person or of life can logically be defined by one of the person's or life's parts. Thus: *'X is bad . . . and therefore I am bad.'* This is known as the part–whole error and is illogical.	**An acceptance belief is logical** An acceptance belief is based on the idea that the whole of a person or of life cannot be defined by one or more of the person's or life's parts. Thus: *'X is bad, but this does not mean that I am bad. I am a fallible human being even though x occurred.'* Here the part–whole illogical error is avoided. Rather, it is held that the whole incorporates the part, which is logical.
A depreciation belief has largely unhealthy consequences A depreciation belief has largely unhealthy consequences because it tends to lead to unhealthy negative emotions, unconstructive behaviour and highly distorted and biased subsequent thinking when you are facing an adversity.	**An acceptance belief has largely healthy consequences** An acceptance belief has largely healthy consequences because it tends to lead to healthy negative emotions, constructive behaviour and realistic and balanced subsequent thinking when you are facing an adversity.

- *'I cannot act differently because I do not feel competent yet.'* As with comfort and control, feelings of competence will come from doing things incompetently and as a result of learning from your errors.

- *'I cannot take new action which is strange to me because I do not feel confident to do so.'* Doing things unconfidently is again the remedy here.

- *'I cannot take constructive actions, particularly those which are risky for me, because I do not have the courage to do so.'* As studies of people who have acted heroically in war have shown, a feeling of courage does not come before actions which are regarded as courageous. Those people who act courageously and those people who don't are equally anxious. The difference is that those people who are prepared to act courageously are not waiting for a courageous feeling to come before they act. So, feel the fear and do it anyway.

Stage 9: Correct distortions about the interpretations you made at Stage 4
If you recall, in Stage 4 of this sequence I asked you to assume temporarily that the conditions that you were facing and that you were disturbed about were true. I did this to encourage you to identify your irrational beliefs which led to your disturbance in the first place. Now is the time to go back and to ask yourself how likely it is that your interpretation was true. What cognitive distortions are you making? In Step 7 of the book, I showed you how to identify various thinking distortions and how to challenge them, and I refer you back to that step at this point. The main reason why I suggest that you do not correct your distortions at Stage 4 of this sequence is that at that point you are still under the influence of your disturbed negative feelings and do not have the necessary objectivity to stand back and check on the accuracy of your interpretation. Questioning your beliefs at Stage 7 helps you to gain such objectivity and encourages you to correct any distortions that remain in your thinking.

Stage 10: Generalize to other relevant situations Once you have gained practice in, say, overcoming your need for approval from people at work, you can then generalize your new rational beliefs (e.g. 'I'd like to have approval, but I don't need it') to other situations where approval may be an issue for you – for example, in your relationships with your parents, spouse or children. Don't assume that such generalization will occur spontaneously. It won't. You need to build it in rather than to wait passively for it to happen.

Stage 11: Maintain your gains You may hold the erroneous idea that once you have benefited from a programme of counselling, or some self-change project, you have achieved your goals and you do not have to work to maintain your gains. However, human beings have a unique talent to lapse and lapse if they do not make a commitment to work consistently to maintain such gains (as anybody who has undertaken to lose weight or to give up smoking will readily testify). If you resolve to practise strengthening your new rational beliefs every day, even though there is no obvious need for you to do so, you will experience the benefits of this later.

In order to minimize the chance that lapses and relapses may happen, you need to plan for them in advance. Look in particular for your vulnerability factors. For example, in trying to minimize your drinking, you may find yourself with friends who like to down six or seven pints. If you are prone to anxiety, your vulnerability factor might be being in unfamiliar situations. The more you can identify your vulnerability factors in advance and the more you can identify, challenge and change the irrational beliefs that lead these to be vulnerability factors, then the more you will minimize the chances of lapsing or relapsing.

Initially, it might be helpful to stay away from vulnerable situations until you have strengthened your rational beliefs to such an extent that you are able to confront them successfully. I don't want you to be in a situation where you feel overwhelmed, but I do want you to develop the habit of challenging yourself in healthy ways. Having said all this, since you are human, lapses will still occur. There is no absolute way to avoid them. If you accept yourself and do not disturb yourself about the existence of lapses, you will be in a much better position to learn from them. However, if you condemn yourself or unduly disturb yourself about a lapse, this will easily turn into a relapse, and although you will not quite be back at square one this is how it may seem to you.

In conclusion, realize that maintaining your mental health involves a lifetime commitment to hard work. The good news is that it does get easier the more you do it. The other good news is that no human being is or can ever be perfectly mentally healthy. Not even me! Good luck!

Index